ALSO BY GENEEN ROTH

Appetites

When Food Is Love

Breaking Free from Compulsive Eating

Why Weight?

Feeding the Hungry Heart

When You Eat at the
Refrigerator, Pull Up a Chair

Fifty Ways to Feel

Thin, Gorgeous, and Happy

(When You Feel

Anything But)

When You Eat

at the Refrigerator,

Pull Up a Chair

Geneen Roth

Foreword by Anne Lamott

NEW YORK

Copyright © 1998, Geneen Roth and Associates, Inc.

Illustrations by Robbin Gourley

Excerpt from "Saint Francis and the Sow" from *Three Books* by Galway Kinnell. Copyright © 1993 by Galway Kinnell. Previously published in *Mortal Acts, Mortal Words* (1980). Reprinted by permission of Houghton Mifflin Company. All rights reserved.

Excerpt from "The Low Road" from *The Moon is Always Female* by Marge Piercy. Copyright © 1980 by Marge Piercy. Reprinted by permission of Alfred A. Knopf, Inc.

Library of Congress Cataloging-in-Publication Data
Roth, Geneen.
     When you eat at the refrigerator, pull up a chair : 50 ways to feel thin, gorgeous, and happy (when you feel anything but) / Geneen Roth; foreword by Anne Lamott — 1st ed.
       p. cm.
     ISBN 0-7868-6395-1
     1. Weight loss — Psychological aspects. 2. Body image. I. Title.
RM222.2.R6674   1998
613.2'01'9 — dc21   97–38725
                                                              CIP

FIRST EDITION

10   9   8   7   6   5   4   3   2   1

For Jeanne Hay,

godmother of my heart

and

Lynne August,

farmer, mentor, friend

Contents

Foreword by Anne Lamott   xi

Note to the Reader Who Does Not Struggle with Food   xvii

Introduction   1

1. Whatever You Do, Don't Diet/9   2. Cultivate
Curiosity/15   3. When You Eat at the Refrigerator,
Pull Up a Chair/20   4. Give Away Clothes That
Cut Off Your Circulation/23   5. Consider Howard
Stern and Live "As If"/27   6. Learn to Recognize
a Fat-and-Ugly Attack/31   7. Emergency
Interventions/36   8. Act On Your Own Behalf/39
9. Eat a Hot Meal Every Day/43   10. Be Fully
Present for Five Minutes Every Day/47
11. Whenever You Feel Fat or Ugly or Worthless, Ask
Yourself Whose Instructions You Are Following/51
12. Do Not Sneak Food or Feelings/57   13. Retail

Therapy Is As Important as the Other Kind/60
14. Learn the Difference Between Self-Indulgence and
Self-Kindness/63   15. Carry a Chunk of Chocolate
Everywhere/67   16. Lose the Muumuus and
Just-in-Case Clothes/73   17. Wear Red/77
18. Begin to Tolerate Joy/81   19. Remember that
Thin People Have Cellulite, Get Old, and Die/84
20. Eat Enough Fat/87   21. Remember that There Is
No Right Way, Right Path, Right Answer, Right
Food/90   22. Wear a Belt/93   23. Three Ways to
Stop a Fat-and-Ugly Attack/94   24. When There
Are Tigers Above You and Tigers Below You, Eat a
Ripe Strawberry/99   25. Stare at Normal Women's
Bodies (Normal Does Not Include Models, Actresses,
and Elite Athletes)/104   26. Wear Your Special-
Occasion Clothes Any Old Day/109
27. More About Presence: The Practice of Sensing Your
Arms and Legs/114   28. No Matter What You've

Consumed in the Past Twenty-four Hours, Twenty-four
Days, or Twenty-four Years, Eat the Very Next Time
You Get Hungry/118   29. . . . And Stop When
You've Had Enough/123   30. Remind Yourself
That It's Already Broken/137   31. Lagniappe/131
32. Develop Friendships That Applaud Your Strengths
and Celebrate Your Successes/134   33. . . . And
Begin to Gently Let Go of Friends Who Don't Want
the Best for You/137   34. Eliminate the Ways You
Gain Weight Without Eating/141   35. When Things
Begin to Fall Apart, Let Them/145   36. Ask for
Help: You Can't Do It Alone/148   37. When You
Are Not Hungry, Beauty Is Better than Bonbons/154
38. Practice Saying No/158   39. Be Willing to Lose
the Suffering Contest/161   40. Eat Enough Protein/165
41. About the Activity Formerly Known as Exercise/169
42. Take the Woo-Woo Out of Meditation/177
43. Burn Your Diet Books in Your Bathtub and Other

Rituals/179   44. Do One Exquisitely Kind Thing
for Yourself Every Day/188   45. When Diets Do
Work/191   46. Consider Resigning from Your
Fondness for Drama/200   47. Food and Your
Mother Go Together/203   48. Separate the Desire to
Be Thin from the Desire to Be Cherished/207
49. Celebrate Every Little Thing/210   50. Decide on
an Everyday Practice and Do It No Matter
What   220

Foreword

Geneen Roth's books amaze me, this new one maybe even more than the others, and that's saying quite a lot. Before I read Geneen's first book, *Feeding the Hungry Heart*, I spent a quarter of a century either on a diet and being good, or falling off the diet and eating my body weight in fats and sugars and carcinogens. I loved being too thin. I loved having people worry about me. "We've got to put a little meat on those bones," they'd say with concern. Words like these made my heart soar. Unfortunately, after a number of years my heart really was soaring—like someone about to have a heart attack as the result of grave electrolytic imbalance.

The madness did not begin to come to an end until February 13, 1987, when I ate three gigantic meals and chased down each with a glass of Epsom salts. Epsom salts were my purging drug of choice—they're the all-time greatest laxative, although there are several unpleasant little side effects: muscle cramps, heart arrhythmia, death. Shaking and totally out of control, I realized I was in serious danger. The next day, I met for the first time with a therapist named Rita who had been reading Geneen's books. I never purged again.

I'm not sure why I want to begin this Foreword to Geneen's deeply nourishing new book with secrets about how damaged I am about food. Maybe so that you will know that I qualify to write food miracles—that I am one of you. That you are one of us. Maybe so that you will believe that if Geneen's gentle birth-coaching can help me break through, it can help anyone.

Geneen's writing has helped me change my life dramatically, helped me find my way home after a lifetime lost on the highways and byways of food obsession. Her books have helped me find freedom after being held hostage by a distorted body image and the values of a culture that I don't actually buy. She takes one of the most complicated and confusing and antagonistic parts of my life — my body and me, my body and food, my weight, my heart, my being — and she renders it clear and compassionate. She gently throws the lights on for me.

I love this new book especially because it is so distilled, so essential. I love it also because it came along during one of the rockiest emotional times of my life. I had just ended a romance with someone I thought I might marry, gone through a gigantic amount of pain and loss, and then found myself crushed because through it all, my weight stayed the same. I felt so ripped off! Usually if I hurt enough emotionally, I drop a few pounds, and then I look gaunt and needy, and everyone feels more tenderly toward me. But I didn't lose any weight when my romance ended, and when I saw how sad this made me, I realized once again that this food thing—this body thing—is so tough.

Until I encountered Geneen's work, I had no sense that I deserved all the miracles that food can be about—nourishment, deliciousness, health. I just thought that if I lost a few more pounds, and maybe started jogging, everything would fall into place. I was convinced that I needed to resist food, that doing so would prove that I was a strong person. I felt that if I tasted and loved the food that went slipping down my throat, then I would be vulnerable to all manners of terrible desire. Also, that I would end up weighing well over 1,200 pounds.

It's been a long road—three steps forward, two steps back. From time to time, I still slip into my old patterns. I wake up some mornings and decide that I absolutely must lose a few pounds, begin a new diet, join a health club, and make an appointment in Rio for a little liposuction. Once a year, I sneak off to the local drug store and—with the furtiveness of someone buying the rankest pornography—buy a cheap bathroom scale. Then, several days later, when the trance has broken, I slink down to the Salvation Army collection center and hand my contraband to the puzzled Asian volunteer who works the collection bin. "Here's another scale," I always say cheerfully. After a long moment, he always replies, "Thanks."

Wherever you are on the path toward health and balance, whether you have just begun the process or are many years along, these essays will guide you, feed you, make you laugh, and provide some light for each day's healing. They will help you understand or remember that everything you need for self-acceptance and joy is inside you now, like seeds already planted in the moist ground of a garden. All it takes for them to grow is a little water, a little time, a little attention, a little love.

The gift of this book is that the pieces are so small and perfectly self-contained. Geneen's richness and wisdom and deep compassion and wonderful humor come to us on such exquisite little plates this time.

So, make yourself a lovely cup of tea, put on your favorite soft pants, wrap yourself in a blanket given to you by someone who loves you, and breathe.

Come join us on the road back.

—Anne Lamott

Note to the Reader
Who Does Not Struggle
with Food

Throughout the book, I have used feelings of being "fat" interchangeably with feelings of being incompetent, unattractive, unworthy, out of control, valueless, invisible. Our culture links fatness with an entire world of undesirable qualities, and unfortunately, women who struggle with their weight do the same.

If you do not identify with the issue of fatness per se, you can substitute anything you don't want to be or feel in its place. Although I am most familiar with feelings of unworthiness as they translate through body size, issues of the heart are universal.

And despite all rumors to the contrary, if you are the kind of person who cannot gain weight no matter what you eat, and who looks at other women in amazement when they talk about sacrificing their firstborn for caramel custard, you are written into these pages just the same.

When You Eat at the

Refrigerator, Pull Up a Chair

Introduction

My loosest jeans are tight on me today. This is not a good sign.

Last week was Passover, the holiday that celebrates the liberation of the Jews from slavery and their exodus from Egypt. We acknowledge this freedom by telling the Passover story at ritual gatherings called seders. We also acknowledge it by consuming astonishing amounts of food that people who are trying to free themselves from strokes and heart attacks wouldn't consider eating.

Last week, I ate matzoh balls made with chicken fat, fruit compote made with pineapples dipped in heavy syrup, and noodle pudding made with butter, brown sugar, and sour cream. For dessert, I ate cheesecake and two kinds of flourless chocolate cake.

Every night for five nights.

During the day, I ate leftovers from the night before.

Although I make it a practice not to weigh myself, my fat jeans tell me I've gained weight, possibly four or five pounds, and, for the umpteenth time, I'm convinced that my brain has truly snapped and I am five minutes away from being as big as a house. Or at least a small cottage.

The way I see it today, I have a few options: liposuction, buying bigger jeans, or flailing myself. Of the three, the only one that is completely out of the question is bigger jeans. (My husband, Matt, suggested the jeans option. He thought it was reasonable. I told him I would rather get a root canal without Novocain. That ended the discussion.) The problem with liposuction is that it goes against every principle I have. Also, besides being costly, it is terribly inefficient as it doesn't account for future Passovers, Thanksgivings, or trips to Bette's Bakeshop for Death-by-Chocolate cake. This leaves flailing myself about being a hypocrite who has written five books on eating disorders, worked with over forty thousand people during the twenty years I've been teaching Breaking Free® from Compulsive Eating workshops, and can now only fit into oversized green flannel pajamas.

Of course, there is another option: disengaging from the alluring drama of feeling fat and its attendant swoops of emotion. (Which is not the same as bingeing or giving up.) Feeling fat is like Krazy Glue; it takes a herculean effort to separate from it. It also takes kindness, curiosity, and a willingness to act on my own behalf—all of which can be learned. But I am quite fond of drama, and learning these things has not come easily. I am most familiar with myself as an insecure, angsting, bingey type of gal who could gain weight or fall apart at the slightest provocation. Replacing this woozy self-image with one of solidity and strength has been, and continues to be, a many-stepped process.

This book is about that process.

In twenty years of observing myself closely and listening to thousands of women talk about the size of their bodies and the size of their lives, I have learned this much: Feeling fat has nothing to do with *being* fat. I've heard women who are a size sixteen talk about how thin they felt, and I've heard women who are a size four talk about how fat they felt. I've also heard women talk about feeling fat one moment and thin the next.

In one of my recent workshops, someone said, "If I woke up tomorrow and this whole issue with food was gone, I wouldn't know how to measure myself. Right now, being thin is how I know I'm good. Feeling fat is how I know I'm bad. If I didn't have this system of fat and thin, I would feel terribly lost." The feeling of fatness has little to do with whether or not you are fat, and everything to do with your identity and self-image, with the particular "flavor" you've come to recognize as your inner world.

We wouldn't resort to feeling fat or ugly or dumb if it didn't serve us in basic, primal ways. Because twenty-five million women in our country are on daily diets, feeling fat keeps us connected to other people as well as being the familiar way we know ourselves. By allowing us to remain active members of the most popular club in the country — those who perpetually struggle with their weight — feeling fat keeps us safe and acceptable.

The problem is that it also cuts us off at the knees. When you feel fat — no matter what you weigh — you take a pair of scissors to your life and cut it down to the size you think it's supposed to be in order for you to be loved and accepted.

Most important, when you tell yourself you feel fat, you make it impossible to figure out what is actually going on. Perhaps you really are uncomfortable with your size and are ready to lose weight. Perhaps you feel lonely or excited or happy or threatened. You will never know what you feel, or what you need to do, as long as you translate uncomfortable or unfamiliar feelings, positive or negative, into the familiar refrain of feeling fat.

For many years, my students have been asking me

to write the kind of book they could carry with them on buses and read in the middle of a dive into cheese nachos. The kind of book they could pick up when they need to be reminded that being thin and happy and gorgeous is just a breath away. For just as feeling fat has nothing to do with the size of your body, neither does feeling thin. Both are shorthand for inner states of mind and heart. While there is obviously a physical reality of fatness or thinness, that reality is profoundly affected by the things we say to ourselves, the lack of respect or curiosity or kindness we are able to muster.

This book is about understanding that what you want from being "thin and gorgeous and happy" will never be achieved by telling yourself you are fat and ugly. It is about understanding that the open-hearted, powerful, expansive state most people associate with being thin is directly connected to, and profoundly influenced by, your inner life. When the women I work with contact that power, strength, and joy inside themselves, they suddenly realize that these are what they wanted all along, what they thought they could get only by being thin. They realize they have everything they want *now;* they are already whole, already complete. After arriving at this understanding, they are no longer fighting the voices in their heads that tell them they are fat and ugly, and simultaneously want to deprive them of the only sweetness left: food. Losing weight is no longer a struggle because the whole of them — their minds and their bodies — is now on the same side.

During the years I've been teaching workshops, students have asked me to repeat certain things over and over. Certain questions are always asked; certain themes always emerge. Everyone wants to know how to remove the obstacles that keep them from realizing their innate strength, power, and joy; they want to know how to lose weight without torturing themselves, how to end the obsession with food, and why chocolate is not a major food group.

These are the things I have written about here. These are the things I say to myself and to the women in my workshops when we are convinced that this time, we not only feel fat, we *are* fat.

May this book help you act on your own behalf with kindness, curiosity, and humor. May it help you free yourself so that everything in your life becomes fluid, unfettered, and easy. Including, of course, your jeans.

1. Whatever You Do, Don't Diet

I've gained and lost over a thousand pounds in my life. I've been anorexic, sixty pounds overweight, and every point in between. I've been on the Atkins Diet; the Prunes and Meatball Diet; the Thousand-Calorie-a-Day Sugar Diet; the Coffee, Diet Creme Soda, and Cigarette Diet; Weight Watchers; and water fasts. All of them worked for a week, a month, even a year. And then every single one of them stopped working.

When you feel fat and ugly, the thought of going

on a diet is incredibly seductive. You watch those breezy, thin women pull out the waist of their pants on the Jenny Craig ads. Or you read the latest article about "Ten Butt Busters to Blast into Bikinis" and you decide that if only you could blast your butt, everything would be fine. A burst of hope fills you with inspiration, energy, willpower. Soon you will be pulling out the waist of your tight jeans. You're going on a diet!

Don't. And this is why:

1. The fourth law of the universe is that for every diet, there is an equal and opposite binge. Diets aren't free. You will rebel, and when you do, you will gain more weight than you lost. As fat as you feel now, you will feel — and be — fatter after the binge that follows the diet.

2. The basic message of a diet is that if you let yourself go, you will devour the universe. But you cannot say anything to yourself physically that doesn't also affect you emotionally. When you diet, you tell yourself that you can't be trusted, that your hunger (for love, pleasure, friendship) will destroy people. You begin to believe you are hopeless, a bottomless pit. This is not a kind thing to say to yourself. It is also not true. No one's hunger is bottomless.

3. Deprivation, fear, shame, and guilt do not now, and never will, lead to long-lasting change. You might desperately want to change, you might be whole-heartedly ready to lose weight. You might be ready to discipline yourself, to be conscious of what, when, and how much you eat. But dieting based on shame, deprivation, and fear is not the way. Beating a child might force her to conform to your wishes, but it will also make her so frightened that her focus will be to avoid another beating, not to understand her motivation or the reasons for it being necessary to change her behavior.

4. Long-lasting change can only come through kindness to yourself, curiosity about what you do, and a willingness to act on your own behalf. Diets are like having a mean, abusive parent inside your head. Diets keep you stuck being a cowering child.

Before we go any further, I want to make something clear: Not dieting does not equal bingeing. Not dieting does not equal going numb or unconscious. I know this is hard to believe. I've received letters from people who tell me they throw my books against the wall, give them to their dogs to eat, or use them for kindling because they are so furious with me for suggesting they can eat what they want. I understand their mistrust; I felt it myself.

When I stopped dieting, I was terrified. Since I had spent every single day for seventeen years on either a diet or a binge, I was certain that given the permission to eat as much ice cream as I wanted, I would devour the entire gallon. But after the initial glee of releasing myself from diet jail, I discovered that it was the forbiddenness itself that made certain foods so attractive; I wanted what I couldn't have. When I gave myself permission to eat a gallon of ice cream without feeling as if I were having a secret affair with a married man, I didn't want it anymore. (Okay, I confess. It took two rounds of eating the whole gallon *without guilt* before I realized that being sick to my stomach was not the way I wanted to spend the evening.) I began to understand that the only reason I had previously wanted the whole thing was because I wouldn't let myself eat even a teaspoonful without guilt. When I took the forbiddenness away, I also took away the need to rebel. When I stopped dieting, I stopped bingeing.

A student of mine was sixty pounds over her natural weight when she first started breaking free from dieting. One rainy winter night, she and her husband were cooking dinner and she realized she didn't want pot roast and vegetables, she wanted a piece of lemon meringue pie from Annie's Place, in town. She sat with her husband while he ate his dinner, and then they drove to Annie's Place, although it was ten miles away. Sloshing into the restaurant, they ordered tea and lemon meringue pie. My student took three bites of the pie and said, "I've had enough." Her husband was incredulous. "We just drove ten miles in the driving rain, and you only want three bites?" She nodded her head and said, "Geneen said we should eat what we want and stop when we've had enough. I've had enough." He finished the pie. She told me later, "It really wasn't the pie I wanted. I wanted to know I deserved to have what I wanted. And I wanted to know I was worth driving ten miles in a storm to get it. Once I did that, the pie was unimportant." She became more and more discriminating about what she wanted to eat, and when; at the end of eight months, she had lost forty pounds. (Her husband, however, couldn't bear leaving food on a plate and gained twenty!)

In *Zen Mind, Beginner's Mind*, Shunryu Suzuki talks about giving farm animals big pastures in which to roam. He says that when you fence them in too tightly, they become wild and restless, but when you provide wide, open spaces, they relax. The same is true of human beings.

Years ago, when I needed to know my mother was telling me the absolute truth, I'd say, "You promise?" And she'd say, "I really, really promise."

Right now, I want you to know that no matter how ugly or fat you feel at this very moment, you can lose weight and keep it off without dieting. I really, really promise.

2. Cultivate Curiosity

Blanche, my cat, is my role model. He never assumes he knows the answer, and he is always prepared for the miraculous. He stalks a brown paper grocery bag as if it could suddenly sprout legs and turn into a bear. His endless curiosity is one of the many reasons I have three portraits of him hanging in my house, although he is wearing his red fez in only one of them.

Remember when you used to be curious? Remember when you used to think anything could happen?

That gnomes lived in forests and tiny people lived in your television set? Somewhere along the line, we decided we knew all the answers. We knew what was supposed to happen, we knew what we needed to change to make it happen, and we knew how to go about making the change. All we had to do was summon a little willpower and slap ourselves into place.

One of my main functions as a teacher is to rekindle a student's interest in herself. To assume that no matter how it may appear, she has good reasons for her behavior, and simply to be curious about what those reasons are. About why she is certain that feeling her pain will cause her to go crazy. About why she believes she needs food to deal with her emotions.

"I eat because I am under stress."

If you gently inquire into this statement, you might realize you believe that feeling stress would rip you apart, and that it is better to be fat than to be ripped apart. But where did you get that idea?

Do you believe that excess weight provides a cushion for you, a protective padding? Does your child's mind believe that with enough weight, you can't get physically or emotionally hurt, that there are too many layers to get through? Do you believe that if you stopped eating, the layers would disappear and you'd be left unprotected or ripped apart?

We have exquisitely good reasons for doing what we do, for believing what we believe. But unless we are actively curious about them, we will never discover what those reasons are. And unless we know what they are, we cannot ask ourselves if they are still true or helpful or protective, if they are as relevant today as when we first developed them.

A student recently told me that she was despairing about her habit of eating when she really needed to be working. "Eating is my way of procrastinating, and it's incredibly self-destructive," she said. "I feel stuck and miserable." I asked her to write a "Curiosity Dialogue" about why she used food to procrastinate.

Afterward she said, "Last year I was very ill because I worked myself into the ground. I don't trust myself to know when to stop. I believe that if I don't procrastinate, I'll do the same thing I did last year and end up very sick. Overeating stops me from working so hard. It is my stop-gap measure, my protection from getting sick again."

Through being curious, she began to understand the motives underlying her overeating. Once she understood the pattern, she realized that she could change. She could set limits for herself; she could be mindful about stopping when she was tired, and getting enough rest. She didn't have to use food to protect herself from getting sick. She could take true care of herself.

The next time you tell yourself you eat because of stress (or depression, anger, sadness, loneliness, etc.), stop. Begin writing an ongoing "Curiosity Dialogue." Keep it in a separate notebook.

Open with simple, declarative statements.

Describe the event that triggered your desire to eat.

Be interested in why you feel what you feel.

Where in your body are your feelings located? What color are they? What texture? What shape?

If you don't know, take a wild guess (i.e., "I have a red ball of anger in the center of my chest. It feels hot and fiery.").

What do you believe would happen if you allowed yourself to feel your feelings instead of avoiding them or swallowing them with food?

Every time you feel stuck, every time you think you know why you are doing something but you can't seem to make yourself do it differently, write a dialogue with yourself.

Assume that you're innately sane and extraordinarily wise. Your job is to ask questions, not to manufacture answers. The answers have been there all the time, sleeping under the brown grocery bag of your broken heart. You just haven't looked.

Be open to the outcome. Predict nothing. Be ready for anything. You will be constantly surprised.

3. When You Eat at the Refrigerator, Pull Up a Chair

ꙮ

Imagine you . . .

Invite a friend over for dinner.

Tell her that the two of you are going to eat the way you eat when you are alone. Explain that you are going to treat her the way you treat yourself: Lead her to the refrigerator. Open the door. Stare.

Begin picking from Tupperware containers. Use your fingers.

Graze through yesterday's Chinese food. Last

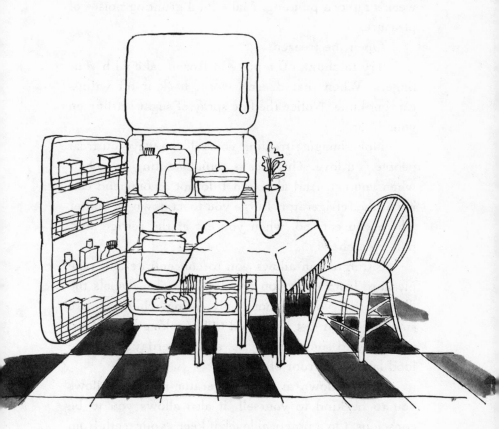

week's tapioca pudding. Make loud grunting noises of pleasure.

Open the freezer.

Try to chunk off a piece of frozen cake with your fingers. When that doesn't work, hack it off with a carving knife. Notice the fine spray of sugar settling on your floor.

Now, imagine treating yourself the way you treat people you love. This means actually sitting in a chair when you eat. And although I do not recommend eating at the refrigerator, I urge you to sit down no matter where you eat. So, when you eat at the refrigerator, pull up a chair.

Sitting down allows you to concentrate and take pleasure from what you are doing. It also dispels the illusion that you are not really eating while you are standing—you just happened to be looking around, on your way to somewhere else, and yesterday's Chinese food landed in front of you.

Sitting down at the refrigerator not only allows you to be kind to yourself, it also allows you to be conscious. On a practical level, it keeps your teeth from being broken by fossilized cake.

4. Give Away Clothes That Cut Off Your Circulation

Almost every woman I know has three sizes of clothes in her closet: thin clothes, fat clothes, and in-between. Fat clothes—"just-in-case clothes"—keep you frightened of gaining weight (see chapter 16), while thin clothes keep you waiting for your life to begin. Thin clothes, the ones you need a shoehorn to shimmy into, are those that cut off your circulation at the waist or arms or thighs.

The possibilities of daily torture, self-recrimination, and warped fantasies are endless when you hang on to clothes that represent a time when you had what you thought you wanted most — a thin body — and for one reason or another, don't have anymore. Why not be kind to yourself and give them away?

Believe me, I know how hard it is. Last year, I finally gave away the dress I wore to an ex-boyfriend's wedding twenty years ago — a navy blue form-fitting gown with pale-blue silk piping and gold frog buttons. The bottom third of the dress was flowing and loose, but the hips and waist were designed to feel like a second skin. Unfortunately, my first skin was fifteen pounds more than it needed to be to fit into the dress. So I did the old "I have to lose twenty pounds to look good at the wedding" number and convinced myself that my excess weight was the reason Steven didn't love me. I dreamed that when the minister asked if anyone could see a just reason why these two people should not be joined together, I would be such a knock-out that Steven would run to my side.

To accomplish this task, I had to go on a meatball, Grape-Nuts, and Mott's Diet Strawberry applesauce diet (I made it up), from which I did not waver for three weeks. Before the ceremony, someone's aunt Riva spilled a Bloody Mary on my dress. Steven married Andrea without a hitch. Later that night, with just the teeniest edge of bitterness and bile, I threw the dress in the washing machine and ate a half gallon of Breyers Vanilla Fudge Twirl ice cream. The next day, I devoured a lemon icebox cake, and within a month, I'd gained back the fifteen pounds. For years after that, I'd try on the too-tight dress and use it as a measuring stick for my failures. Somehow I managed to convince myself that if only I could fit into that dress again, I'd be happy, loved, content.

The truth is, of course, that Steven wouldn't have loved me no matter what I weighed. I know this because he is still married to Andrea and she recently called my office and asked to come to an intensive class because she'd gained sixty pounds. (A better person than I am would not be happy by this turn of events.) In any case, just looking at the dress in my closet for the past twenty years made me feel like a fat, ugly sloth. The fantasy I'd constructed around it—and my too-tight leggings, as well as the gray pantsuit I bought after I had the flu one year and hadn't eaten for two weeks—were keeping me from getting on with my life.

Thin clothes scream obscenities at you:

"You idiot. How could you let yourself go?"

"Remember when you slid right into these pants? Life was good then. You were thin then. You dropped the ball, sister. Suck in your stomach, shut your mouth, stop eating like a crazed lunatic and lose some weight!"

Thin clothes tell you that you are out of control and that your life will be better when you slap yourself back into shape. They keep you panting for a time in the future when you will be allowed to enjoy yourself again. Most of all, they tell you that who you are now is definitely NOT ACCEPTABLE.

Get rid of them. You have enough mean, abusive voices in your head without having to hang them in your closet.

Replace them with clothes that fit you now. Clothes that are soft and luscious and allow you to feel the same.

5. Consider Howard Stern and Live "As If"

ꙮ

This is what I find interesting about Howard Stern: He's a famous shock jock with two best-selling books, a movie made about his life, and every dream come true. Yet he still feels like garbage. He reminds me of the women in my classes who stand up and say, "I lost fifty pounds and I still feel fat and ugly and miserable."

In an article in the *New Yorker*, Stern's producer, Robin Quivers, said, "Howard is constantly revisiting the past and somehow it isn't enough to have the whole world be in love with him. He still wants the people who didn't love him before to love him now. A couple of weeks ago, we were on the phone with some girl he had wanted but she'd dated a friend of his instead. Howard called her up and said, 'See who I am now? Look at what a great life you could have had. I would have married you.' He really wants them to feel how wrong they were. And it has to be somebody who 'knew me then, didn't love me then. I want to hear them love me now.' And he's never going to get that. Because they don't love him. They didn't love him then and they don't love him now."

In the same article, Stern said, "I always feel like garbage. I could go to a book signing and see twenty thousand people out there and I don't feel great from that. You'd think that kind of adulation would make you feel on top of the world. And yet I don't. I don't know why."

I hear variations on this theme from my students all the time. "When I get thin, everyone who didn't love me before will love me then. When I get thin, I will be happy. Everything will be wonderful." And then they get thin, and the people who didn't love them before still don't love them, and even worse, they are still not happy. Being thin has not changed anything except the size of their bodies. Often, they feel so let down that they turn to food again to comfort themselves. And the cycle continues.

Being thin is a body size. A body size cannot give you love. We give magical power to thinness, and then believe we need the thinness to get the power back. But the power was ours to begin with; the joy, the self-worth, the strength, the fulfillment are internal, not external, states. They have nothing to do with what you weigh on a scale, as anyone will tell you who has lost weight and still feels fat.

To change your internal feeling of fatness, you must change how you see yourself, what you give yourself, what you believe you deserve. It is not difficult, but it does take time. It takes kindness and curiosity and acting on your own behalf. It takes putting your insights into action.

A simple, direct way of acting with kindness on your own behalf is living "as if." As if you deserve everything that you believe only size-four women deserve. As if putting roses on your dresser, wearing soft, silky clothes, and sitting down at the table instead standing up at the refrigerator is natural to you. As if you are someone who is worthy of joy and being cherished. When you live "as if," you'll hear a voice inside shouting, "YES! I do deserve, YES! I will sit down, YES! I am gorgeous."

And you will be right.

6. Learn to Recognize a Fat-and-Ugly Attack

Last Thursday, I received some bad news about several projects I'd been working on, I fought with a friend, and my jeans were tight. By the end of the day, I'd convinced myself that my legs were as fat as tree trunks, my eyes were too close together, Matt was on the brink of death, and I would be forever alone if he died because no other sane person could possibly love me. For a brief moment, there seemed only one thing to do: eat. Then I realized that I was in the throes of a major fat-and-ugly attack.

The problem was that I wasn't aware of the source of the attack, I was only aware of its effects—feeling fat, feeling desperate, wanting to eat. But I decided that rather than spend time figuring out where it all started, I should just stop the damage as soon as I could. So I told the internal critic to shut up and began to act "as if." As if compassion were invented so that I could shower myself with it at this very moment. As if I were brilliant and valuable. As if everything that was worth having was inside my chest.

It worked. Within ten minutes, I felt like a human being again. Only then could I actually be objective about what had happened: what I did to upset my friend, the elements of my projects that didn't work, and why my jeans felt tight.

We usually react to self-attacks in one of three ways:

1. We collapse.

2. We vow to improve ourselves.

3. We get angry and defensive.

The part of our psyche that launches fat-and-ugly attacks is a blend of judgmental aspects of voices from parents, teachers, siblings, lovers, society. It tells us there is only one right way to look, behave, talk, and dress, and that we're doing it the wrong way. We needed these voices to develop. We needed to know that going near a hot stove was going to hurt us; we needed to internalize morals and a code of integrity. In its original form, this internal monitor was designed to protect us and keep us safe. Now, it is the greatest single barrier to change because it shames us into believing we shouldn't be unique, we shouldn't express ourselves. We shouldn't do or say or have anything or be any way our parents or teachers or siblings or culture don't want us to.

Fat-and-ugly attacks happen so quickly, and are usually so unconscious, that recognizing them entails working backward: "Oh, I get it—in the past hour I've gone from feeling fine to feeling very, very small. I must be attacking myself for something." When you suddenly feel as if your stomach is an ever-expanding blob or you are a selfish wretch, it is usually a sign that an attack has taken place. To test this theory, you can ask yourself what has changed in the past seventy-two hours. Or seventy-two minutes. The answer will most often be, You felt criticized or blamed or threatened (by someone else or yourself); it can also be that you felt happy or powerful (see chapter 18).

Familiarize yourself with your habitual mode of reacting to attacks. When you feel threatened or criticized or blamed: Do you suddenly feel as if every single thing about you is wrong? Do you feel small? Do you agree with the attack ("I shouldn't be happy"; "I shouldn't have shown her I loved her"; "I shouldn't have eaten that piece of cheese") and vow that next time, you will get it right? Do you find yourself justifying everything you have said to a particular person in the past week while having images of tying cement blocks on her feet and taking her for a swim?

The very act of recognizing the effects of an attack and naming your preferred mode of reaction — "This feeling of worthlessness is a sign that an attack has taken place; it is not the truth" — will help you disengage from it. Naming what you do causes an instant separation between the action itself and the part of you that names it. It allows you to see that you and the attack are not synonymous, and in that moment, a veil drops. Feelings of restriction are replaced with spaciousness and clarity and light. You suddenly feel whole again.

In perhaps such a revelatory moment, Walt Whitman said, "I am much larger and better than I thought. I did not think I held so much goodness." When you recognize an attack for what it is, you restore yourself to the knowledge of your own goodness. After that, not even sticks and stones can harm you.

7. Emergency Interventions

In the middle of a fat-and-ugly attack, I sometimes feel like a crumpled five-year-old who has lost her ability to reason; mustering the mature voice that disengages from the attack with humor or compassion (see chapter 23) seems impossible. So, I have an "Emergency Interventions" list posted on my refrigerator (next to the sign that says "It's Not in Here") to act as my brain and heart when I feel as if I don't have either.

Doing one or all of the following things when you feel fat will put distance between you and the belief that what you are attacking yourself about is the whole truth:

- ❧ Instead of wearing old, baggy, stained clothes, wear soft, silky fabrics. Choose one article of clothing in your closet that makes you feel royal, elegant, graceful. Put it on. It doesn't matter if it's a batik rayon jacket and you're washing the dishes or picking up your child at nursery school. What matters is that you break the barrage of insults by treating yourself as if you are gorgeous now.

- ❧ Listen to an album of harpist Georgia Kelly or the sound track of the movie *Il Postino*. Both are enveloping, regenerating, and soothing.

- ❧ Take a nap. Take a bath. If you are in the middle of a workday, take a five-minute break.

- ❧ Breathe. It always helps to breathe.

- ❧ Go outside. If you can't go outside, look out a window.

- ❧ Notice the roses; they're still beautiful. They

don't think you are fat. If you can't look at a rose, imagine one. If it's the middle of winter, notice the sky. Remember that the gray is covering a true, endless blue.

Be fierce and tender at the very same time. Fierce in your efforts to stop the attack, and tender with yourself when you do.

8. Act On Your Own Behalf

Acting on your own behalf is a tricky concept for those of us who have spent large portions of our lives on diets. Since, as previously stated, the fourth law of the universe is that for every diet there is an equal and opposite binge, those of us who have dieted have also spent large portions of our lives on binges.

Our experience of acting on our own behalf is that we can't.

Our experience is that no matter what we tell ourselves about the amount and kind of food we are going to eat, about how much we are going to exercise, about how much weight we are going to lose, something always happens and we don't keep our promise to ourselves. We sabotage our plans. We lose faith in our abilities to truly care for ourselves, to take action that fosters our well-being, that feeds our joy, exuberance, vitality, and mental and physical health.

But precisely because diets inevitably lead to binges, the proof you use to tell yourself how weak-willed you are is not valid. It's like saying, "If one and one equals two, then I am a wimp."

You need to learn that you really can—and will—take care of yourself, that you won't leave yourself when things get difficult. That there is someone home inside your body, an adult who knows how to be appropriately kind or firm.

When you practice acting on your own behalf, start with activities that are achievable, not diets whose failure is already a given. Begin with concrete activities that you know you can do, like being on time or remembering to bring something to a friend that you promised to bring. Then follow these five steps:

1. Write down your intention on a piece of paper.

2. Post it where you can see it.

3. Know that it takes effort to change any habitual pattern.

4. Be willing to try.

5. Keep trying.

I used to be ten minutes late for everything. I always had a good excuse: My cat Blanche threw up on the white rug; I got a phone call from Australia; my right side hurt and I had to rest for five minutes just in case I was getting appendicitis. But the real reason was that I never left enough time to get ready. There was something about madly rushing that made me feel important, but it also made me a careless, mean driver, and tied my stomach in knots. After thirty years of being late, I finally realized this year that the edge of excitement and importance that I received from being late was not worth it. I was not acting on my own behalf. I wrote down my intention on a piece of paper—"Leave early. Arrive on time"—and posted it on my desk. After three months of forcing myself to stop whatever I was doing ten minutes before I wanted to stop, I have begun to arrive not just on time, but at gatherings *early*. Change really is possible!

Acting on your own behalf is about doing what you say you are going to do. Not because you will get in trouble if you don't, but because every time you eat when you are not hungry, every time you break a promise to yourself or someone else, you let yourself down. Acting on your own behalf is about slowly becoming a person you can count on. It is about recognizing what you do that causes you pain, and acting on those insights.

Most of all, when you act on your own behalf you stop the war inside yourself. The three-year-old who wants to eat everything in sight stops sabotaging the adult who wants to wire her mouth shut. They both move over to the same side—your own.

time goes on. Two hours later, you are eating a bowl of stale popcorn with spoonfuls of peanut butter, cold hot fudge, and slices of cheddar cheese. Not a winning combination, but it's late and you don't want to take the time to cook a meal. Besides, eating at night is not supposed to be good for you, so all you're going to take is one more bite.

If your life is arranged so that you don't have time to eat a hot meal every day—even if it's soup or scrambled eggs, even if it's vegetable potpie heated in the microwave—it's time to question your priorities.

Most women are so busy providing nourishment for everyone else—children and spouses and friends—that they leave the dregs for themselves. When you don't have a built-in way of giving time and attention to yourself, food becomes the main source of sweetness in your life. And "treats" are usually cold.

Diet sodas, salads, cookies, chips, protein bars, or frozen yogurt are not food. Neither, although hot, is coffee.

You have to start somewhere. You have to begin to be your own advocate, not just with food, but in all

9. Eat a Hot Meal Every Day

Hot meals are real food. Hot meals nourish you. A Snickers bar tastes good, but after you've finished it, you don't feel as if you've eaten. So you go scrounging around for more. Soon you find yourself standing in your kitchen eating three-day-old cold pizza. Then, although it's now ten P.M., you notice the breakfast remains of the french toast your child had for breakfast, and you eat that, too. Still not satisfied, you hunt for more food, and become less and less discriminating as

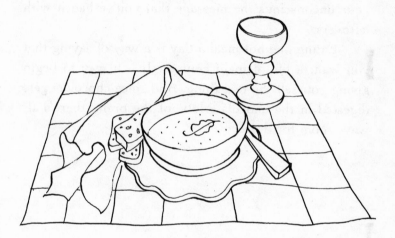

aspects of your life. You have to decide that there's a bottom line, that you have basic needs, and that they are not negotiable. While it's tempting to view a hot meal as a luxury, it's not. One hot meal a day is a basic necessity. Not only to nourish your body, but to give your unconscious the message that you've had it with leftovers.

Eating one hot meal a day is a way of saying that you want a life of main courses. It is a way to begin giving yourself the real thing. And since chocolate gets digested in the chocolate lobe of the brain, there's always room for dessert.

10. Be Fully Present for Five Minutes Every Day

When I first heard the Buddhist description of hungry ghosts—beings in hell with stomachs as big as caves and throats as narrow as pins who live with the perpetual feeling of "not enough"—I was positive I was going straight to hell as a hungry ghost. After all, this was an exact description of my experience with food. And not just with food, with life.

After years of being haunted by this image, I think I've figured out what the hunger is about.

It's about missing my own life.

It's about having food—both physical and emotional—right in front of me, and not being able to taste it because my attention is somewhere else.

We're all walking around hungry for an elusive something, and missing the very thing that could fill us—*showing up*. Being fully present in our own lives.

My friend James, frequently a curmudgeon and always a successful businessman, told me of an astonishing realization: When he was actually aware of lifting his foot while he was lifting his foot, he was completely happy. "I mean the kind of happy I only thought I could be if the deal I am working on comes through next week. I mean the kind of happy that gives happiness its good name."

James was talking about showing up for his own life. He was talking about a quality that you already have because you are born with it—it is called presence, and it happens when all the pieces of you show up where you already are.

Every day we open our eyes, get out of bed, brush our teeth, eat breakfast, talk to our families, do our work. And most of the time, our minds are somewhere else. When we get out of bed, we are thinking about something we should have done yesterday. When we talk to our children, we are thinking about the phone call we need to make. When we walk to the bathroom, we are thinking about the candy we shouldn't have eaten. Or want to eat. Or are going to eat. Or how great our lives are going to be when we lose weight, or get a promotion, or fall in love. Every day, in every moment, we spend our lives thinking about what we already did or are going to do, and we completely miss what we *are* doing. It's like eating a fabulous meal while talking on the phone or watching television. The meal ends and you didn't taste a thing because your attention was somewhere else.

This lack of attention leads to a tremendous hunger that we can't quite name, so we get fooled into thinking that it's for something we don't have yet instead of something that is unfolding minute by minute, right in front of our eyes.

It's almost palpable, that sense of mountainlike solidity that comes with having all your attention on whatever you are doing, whether you are lifting your foot or washing the dishes or playing with your child. Since you are going to do those things anyway — since you have to get out of bed, walk to the bathroom, make breakfast, eat, clean the house — why not be there while you are doing it?

For five minutes a day, bring your full attention to whatever you are doing. Walk while you walk. Talk while you talk. Eat while you eat.

But as with everything else, don't be unreasonably strict with yourself. A famous Zen story describes a teacher who told his students to put their full attention on whatever they were doing, one thing at a time. They practiced hard. They ate while they ate and read while they read. One day, they noticed that the teacher was eating breakfast and reading the newspaper. A brave student approached him, bowed, and said, "Teacher, you tell us to walk while we walk and talk while we talk. But we notice that while you eat, you read." The teacher nodded his head and said, "When you eat, eat, and when you read, read, but when you eat and read, eat and read."

11. Whenever You Feel Fat or Ugly or Worthless, Ask Yourself Whose Instructions You Are Following

During a recent workshop in St. Louis, I was speaking about the importance of questioning and challenging the instructions we receive from our families, the ones we still follow. A woman named Amy jumped up and bolted for the door. I motioned to one of the support counselors to follow her as she ran from the room. A few minutes later, the counselor returned and told me that Amy refused to talk. At the break, I saw her sitting on the couch by herself, smoking a cigarette.

"Is there anything I can help you with?" I asked.

"No. I came here with my daughter. Eating is her problem, not mine, and I just want to be left alone."

"Mind if I sit here with you?" I said.

"You can do anything you want," she said.

We sat there in silence for a few minutes. Then she looked at me and said, "My mother didn't notice my accomplishments, and my father is dead, so there's nothing to be done."

"What happens when *you* notice your accomplishments?" I asked.

"I feel as if I'm not allowed. My mother told me it was wrong to brag."

"Is that why you ran out of the room? Because I was asking you to feel good about something your mother told you was wrong?"

"I ran out because it's too late. My mother still doesn't notice what I do, and my father is dead," she repeated.

"But what about *you* noticing what you do? What about not listening to your mother anymore?"

"Forget it. It's too late."

"Okay, but before I go back in the room, I just want to point out that by sitting here, you are following your mother's instructions to a tee. You'd rather leave the class and sit here by yourself than disobey her."

She glared at me. Then she popped up and shouted, "I WILL NOT!" and went running back into the room. With tears in her eyes, Amy told the rest of the group what had happened. "I know it's not a matter of just deciding I won't listen to her," she said. "I know this will take practice, but I also see for the first time in my life that what my mother said might not have been the truth."

Feeling fat, incompetent, and worthless are the ways most of us stay connected to our families, even if we live three thousand miles away or are eighty-five years old. We learn at an early age what we are allowed to do and who we are allowed to be in relation to the people from whom we need love, and we usually follow these instructions for the rest of our lives.

"Stop being so full of yourself."

"Keep your anger to yourself."

"If you let them see how happy you are, they'll feel bad about their own lives. You don't want people being jealous of you."

"Better not speak up. Better not let them know how you really feel. No one likes bossy, know-it-all girls."

When, as children, the people around us were depressed or angry or lonely, we learned that being joyful or feeling good about ourselves was not a great idea. Not if we wanted to be loved.

For many of us, therefore, allowing ourselves to even recognize (not to mention celebrate) our accomplishments and good fortune feels dangerous. So dangerous that we censor our happiness the very instant we feel it, and replace it with the familiar nonthreatening ways we've come to know ourselves: as always struggling, as fat and ugly and miserable. To most of us, letting go of these self-images feels as if we are three years old and are being asked to let go of our mothers and fathers. Scared to death of being alone, we insist on defining ourselves in reference to our historical families, no matter how old we are. Not because we are juvenile or masochistic, but because we want to be loved and safe and know who we are.

Keep an ongoing list of the instructions you obey or feel guilty about not obeying. This list will include instructions about having too much, about being too happy, about what you need to do to make and keep friends. Remember that these instructions are usually so embedded in your unconscious that you take them to be the truth. Just becoming aware enough to write down these instructions is the first step toward disengaging from them.

Another way of approaching this is to consider the beliefs you have about your life. Beliefs about what is allowed to be easy and what needs to be a struggle. Beliefs about beauty, about clothes, about people who have what they want. All these are shaped by the environment in which you were raised. Unless you examine them and make conscious choices about which ones fit your life now, you will continue to live either in obedience to or in reaction against the set of instructions given to you at the age of three.

The most painful thing about these instructions is

that they diminish your capacity for joy and keep you in the dark about who you really are.

You can take back your life. Suffering is not noble. Feeling fat won't keep you safe. You are allowed to jump for joy.

1 2 . Do Not Sneak
Food or Feelings

Here's what's painful about sneaking:

Every time you sneak food, you give yourself the message that you cannot be seen. You tell yourself, "If they really saw me, they wouldn't love me. Therefore I must hide. Therefore I must sneak." Since you cannot say anything to yourself on a physical level that does not affect you emotionally, sneaking potato chips into your bedroom and eating them under the covers translates to sneaking your desires, sneaking your hungers, sneaking your heart. It perpetuates the belief that who you are is unlovable, too intense, and must be hidden.

Sneaking feelings means not telling the truth.

Count the lies you tell in a day—the times you say you don't care when you do, the times you profess emotion when you feel nothing, the times you add just the slightest twist to a story. You will be shocked at how much you omit, distort, exaggerate, or otherwise change the truth to fit what you perceive to be the needs of the moment. Lying about your actions or your feelings has the same effect as sneaking food. It is a clear message to yourself that you are too much. Too overwhelming. Too powerful. Too petty. Too ruthless. Too strong. Too smart. Too intense. The result of all these lies is that after a while, you can't find yourself. You forget what's really true. And you begin to feel fake because you know that what other people are seeing and loving is not you.

Every time you lie, even if it's a little "white" lie, notice the effect it has on your psyche. Make a commitment to yourself that once a day, you will tell the truth when you ordinarily would have lied, either by eating what you really want in front of whomever happens to be there, or by speaking the truth when you otherwise would have adorned it. Tell someone they've hurt your feelings or that you think the joke they just told was mean, even though everyone else laughed. It doesn't have to be an immense, heart-stopping confrontation; just speaking the truth takes courage.

Do not begin this practice by confessing lies you have told for thirty years or making statements you know will be harmful to other people.

Do not eat in front of people who criticize the size of your body at every opportunity.

Do this with people who already love you.

The reason to tell the truth is to be kind to yourself, and part of being kind to yourself is being able to discriminate between the people who love you and those who don't.

13. Retail Therapy Is As Important as the Other Kind

A few weeks ago, I heard a man on the radio praise shopping. I swear. He said that shopping is the modern version of going to the marketplace. It's the way we see each other, get a feeling for each other, feel included in the social fabric.

My interpretation of his comments is that going shopping is a contemporary equivalent of hunting for moose. We hunt for bargains instead.

I used to think it was wrong to like shopping. That

it was impossible to be wise and also like going to the makeup counter at Nordstrom's. That I couldn't appreciate a good meditation and a good pair of shoes in the same lifetime. I might have gotten this idea from the days when my mother and I, after a satisfying day of being in the marketplace, would tiptoe into the house, enlist my brother as a decoy to occupy my father's attention, and then hide all our packages under my bed. Or from my uncle Leo, who once said, "I'd rather get my bunions scraped than be dragged off to a store by your aunt Janet." Or from my husband, who can't imagine why anyone would rather spend Sunday afternoon wandering around a sweater sale than watching the 49ers with his friends (What could he be thinking?).

In our culture, shopping is classified as a woman's activity, a politically bankrupt form of social behavior. But if grunting and hooting while watching the 49ers is on the list of socially acceptable forms of engagement, I suggest that running your fingers across silky velvets and trying on feathered hats be added to that list. If shopping gives you pleasure, if you do not harm yourself or anyone else while you do it, if it helps you actualize your unique brand of gorgeous, I believe it is worth doing.

Shopping gets you into the world of color, textures, fragrances. You don't have to buy anything. But you can touch everything. You can revel in the variety of fabrics, you can appreciate the display of objects. All your senses can be used when you shop — hearing, seeing, smelling, tasting, touching.

If you don't like to shop, there is no reason to develop a fondness for it. But if you do, allow yourself to enjoy the parade of color and shapes. Be grateful that you don't have most of it cluttering up your house. And when you find a bargain, take pride in your skills. A good moose is hard to find.

14. Learn the Difference Between Self-Indulgence and Self-Kindness

People often mistake tenderheartedness for indulgence, as if being kind to themselves leads to lethargy — sitting around the house all day eating bonbons and wearing muumuus and pink rollers. This is simply not true. I often hear a variation on this statement: "If I'm not intolerant of my shortcomings, how can I ever expect to change them?" And the answer is, By doing the opposite of what you think you need to do to change. By being kind to yourself.

For the record, self-indulgence is

꙲ continuing to do what is harmful to you after you realize it is harmful

꙲ loathing yourself

꙲ getting lost in fantasies about how great your life is going to be while you continue doing the same old self-destructive things

꙲ not asking for help when you need it

꙲ breaking the commitments you've made to yourself

Self-kindness is

꙲ stopping doing what is harmful to you

꙲ defending yourself against anyone who attacks you — including yourself

꙲ telling the truth

꙲ asking for help

꙲ resting when you need rest

꙲ believing that there is a good reason for what

you are doing, even if you aren't aware of it at the moment

From childhood, we are thoroughly conditioned to believe that change can happen only through force. We learn very early to mistrust our intentions. We believe that if we give ourselves enough rope, we will hang ourselves. Karen Russell weighed 424 pounds when I met her. "Telling me I could trust myself with food or feelings was like handing an ax to an ax murderer. That's how I got myself into this mess," she said. "No," I replied, "you got yourself into this mess by not trusting yourself. By repeatedly depriving yourself and then bingeing. After enough binges, you felt like you could devour the universe. Who would trust a gallon of ice cream with anyone who could devour the universe?"

Within a few months of practicing self-kindness — telling her family they were not allowed to comment on her weight, spending time by herself every day, eating exactly what she wanted — she got the hang of it. She started losing weight. Eventually, she treated herself with such kindness that she lost 300 pounds.

In *Lovingkindness: The Revolutionary Art of Happiness,*

Sharon Salzberg writes that we seem to believe that "if we abuse our minds enough with self-hatred and self-condemnation, somehow that abuse will be a path that liberates us. . . . [but] generosity coming from self-hatred becomes martyrdom. Morality born of self-hatred becomes rigid repression. Love for others without the foundation of love for ourselves becomes a loss of boundaries, codependency, and a painful and fruitless search for intimacy."

The only way to learn the difference between self-indulgence and self-kindness is to experience firsthand what self-kindness actually feels like. You learn by going slowly, gently. And you learn by not only reading about, but actually doing the suggestions in this book. Any place is a fine place to begin.

15. Carry a Chunk of Chocolate Everywhere

If you don't like chocolate, please don't feel as if you need to develop a passion for it now. (My husband, Matt, doesn't like chocolate. He has many other lovable qualities, however, and I am certain you do as well.) But if the existence — not to mention the taste — of chocolate is one of the ways you know that ecstasy is available on a daily basis, I offer the following wisdom from years of chocolate education and appreciation.

First, carry your favorite chocolate with you at all

times. Don't depend on restaurants or other people's definitions of good chocolate. I have been shocked and dismayed at what even my best friends consider good chocolate. Devil's food cake with marshmallow filling and gooey icing. Milk chocolate with raisins and nuts. Treats with names like the Seven Dwarfs or Santa's Helpers. Hi-Hos. Ring-Dings. Yodels. If you want to make sure that you get the kind of chocolate you prefer, slip it in your pocket, your purse, your eyeglass case. Don't leave home without it.

Second, don't be ashamed to eat it in public; you never know where it might lead. A few months ago, a television producer asked to interview me for a show he was developing. We met for dinner, and at the end of our meal, I whipped out my purse, pulled out the bar of bittersweet chocolate, broke off a square, and offered him one. His mouth, which had been hanging open since the chocolate first appeared, closed in time to say yes, he would like a piece. We shared a silent moment of ecstasy as the chocolate melted on our tongues, then I put the bar back into my purse, and we proceeded with the meeting. A week later, he called and told me he would like me to appear on his show. "I liked you before you took out the chocolate," he said, "but that clinched it. Anyone who speaks about weight loss, eats chocolate every day, and stays thin knows something other people deserve to know."

What I know is that things, tastes, people, and activities that give you pleasure are good. Not everything that tastes good is bad for you. Chocolate has a place in your life, but like any relationship, you need to pay attention to it.

My third principle of chocolate wisdom is, therefore, "Suck, don't chew." Take time with chocolate. If you pop it in your mouth while you are driving, reading, watching television, feeding your children, talking on the phone, you will keep reaching for more. Soon you will finish the whole bag or box or bar. You will have missed the taste because you were not fully present. You will believe that chocolate and you have a dysfunctional relationship and cannot be in the same room together any longer.

In my workshops, chocolate appreciation begins with Hershey's kisses. Students hold a kiss in their

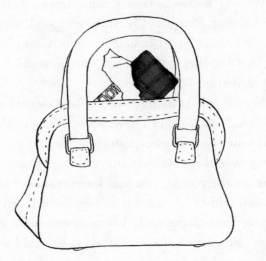

hands, smell it, rub it on their lips, savoring every part of the experience. When they place it in their mouths, they pay close attention to how the taste unfolds. To the explosion of sensation on their lips, tongues, throats. To the difference between sucking on a piece of chocolate and inhaling it. Two or three rapturous minutes pass. They open their eyes, astonished. They can't believe what happens when they pay attention to what they love (a lesson with a wide variety of applications). "One little piece of chocolate tastes so big," they say. They've never eaten just one. The one in their mouths was always merely a precursor to the one they were reaching for, and the ten more after that. Some of them say they thought they were going to love the taste, but are shocked to find that it's too waxy. Others say it's too bland, and they prefer bittersweet chocolate. Still others say if anyone had ever told them they would be satisfied with one kiss, they wouldn't have believed it, but they actually don't want another.

One final chunk of chocolate wisdom: Bring enough to share. Trust me, no matter what is going on at the table before you take out your chocolate, the tone will instantly change when you unveil the wrapper. Conversations will stop. Eyes will gleam. People who didn't notice you before will suddenly find you scintillating. When you share your chocolate, a ripple of excitement infects the gathering. You become everyone's friend.

Chocolate reminds us to wake up, pay attention, stop reaching for what we don't have, and focus on what we do have. It teaches us that we don't need a truck full of love to satisfy our hungry hearts. When we pay attention, enough is possible, here, now, right this very moment.

There are many doors to wisdom. Why not choose one that tastes like shooting stars?

16. Lose the Muumuus and Just-in-Case Clothes

My friend Jesse keeps size fourteen dresses in her closet from the time, fifteen years ago, when she was thirty-five pounds larger than she is now. I call them her just-in-case clothes.

"Who knows when I will suddenly be struck with a mad desire to eat fried sweet potatoes and onion rings, and be unable to stop?" she exclaims.

I tell her that it is possible to eat fried sweet

potatoes and not gain thirty-five pounds. I also tell her that keeping those clothes in her closet keeps fear in her closet. It keeps mistrust in her closet. It keeps her believing that her present state — one of relative stability with food — is only temporary and that with one wrong move, she could feel crazed and numb and out of control again. It keeps her believing that being crazed and numb and out of control is the way she really is, and everything else is pretend.

Keeping muumuu-like apparel in your closet after you have lost weight keeps you believing that you are an impostor in your own life. You wake up every day and see the proof in front of your eyes — the elastic-waist stretch pants, the tentlike dresses. Just-in-case clothes function to keep you off balance just enough so that you never feel confident, never feel grounded in the present moment. If they could talk, they would say, "Who do you think you are, pretending that your life could be the way you want it to be? You are just one step away from disaster, and don't ever forget it."

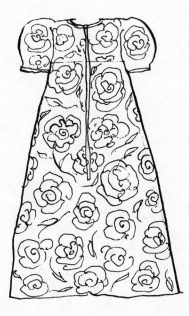

Get rid of the just-in-case clothes; the gesture will be a signal to your unconscious mind that it's time to get rid of the message as well. Neither one of them — the muumuus or the message — is your friend.

1 7. Wear Red

In my opinion, bad-hair days don't hold a candle to feeling-fat days. You open your eyes in the morning and feel sick to your stomach. Then you remember last night's dinner: fried onion rings, pizza with pepperoni and four kinds of cheese, and bread pudding with orange sauce for dessert. (Was there anything green on your plate? You can't recall.)

You sit up and gaze at the middle of your body. A new groundswell of flesh is drifting toward the fluffy area that used to be your stomach. You haul your legs out of bed, and as you waddle to the bathroom, your thighs rub together. You catch a glimpse of yourself in the mirror. Your eyes are slightly swollen, your wrinkles have procreated during the night, and your skin is lackluster from a lifetime of not drinking eight glasses of water a day. Only ten minutes have passed since you woke up.

On bad-hair days, you can wear hats, but since body bags are not an option for feeling-fat days, you have to find an alternative way of putting yourself together. Since you've already given away your muumuus (see chapter 16), and since feeling-fat days call for special-occasion clothes (see chapter 26), the question is, How do you decide which of your special clothes to put on? Is it time for the gold sequins? The purple palazzo pants? The butterfly jacket? The answer is, Wear red.

Over the years, I've learned that certain colors correspond to specific universal qualities. Red corresponds to courage, strength, autonomy, and power. Green corresponds to compassion and a melting heart. Yellow corresponds to joy. As I've experimented with using color as medicine, I've discovered that red is a remarkable antidote for feeling-fat days.

Only yesterday, I was feeling grumpy, pudgy, and tired. I took off the beige shirt I was wearing, and slipped on a red turtleneck instead. Just looking at it lifted my spirits. It wasn't an instant cure, but it reminded me that strength and power were qualities I already possessed, qualities so near that I wear them on my sleeve.

My mother says, "Red is a happy color." Red broadcasts energy, enthusiasm, passion. It also evokes courage and the ability to separate from what's keeping you stuck, which is an important thing to do on a fat day. As I've previously mentioned, feeling fat has very little to do with last night's bread pudding, and everything to do with what meditation teacher Stephen Levine calls "the top-fifty hit parade" of old beliefs. Beliefs about the connection between fat and self-worth, between the size of our bodies and what we are allowed to do or say or be.

Wearing red supports the idea that your past does not rule your life. It is a message to your psyche that says, "Though I ate bread pudding last night, and my stomach is awash with ripples today, I am still allowed to be strong and powerful. I am still allowed to be loved. So, PIPE DOWN!"

P.S. If you've avoided everything red since your flannel pajamas with feet and a flap because you are convinced that wearing red makes you look jaundiced or terminally ill, the word on the street (next to Bloomingdale's) is that with the proper shade of red, anyone's skin will glow. Consider magenta, burgundy, auburn, or ruby. Consider shades that sound like romance novels: Cherries in the Snow, Forever Berry, Russet Moon. But if you are steadfast in your anti-red stance, or if you need to wear sober uniforms to work, remember that you can adorn your toes, nails, and lips with red. As those who have spent years in retail therapy know, the operative word is "accessorize."

1 8. Begin to Tolerate Joy

It came as a shock to me a few years ago that every time I felt joy, I ate great quantities of carob malt balls, and that within an hour or so of feeling joyful, I would be miserable. My misery would sound something like this: "I can't believe you did that. I can't believe you ate half a pound of carob malt balls when you weren't hungry. At least you could have eaten that bittersweet chocolate from Belgium. Or gone for a walk. Or called a friend, or *done anything* but eat malt balls. Not only are you fat, but you also have incredibly poor taste in food."

Ah, the familiar refrain. The familiar attacks. After tracking my bouts into carob treats for about six months, I began to discern the pattern: Something wonderful would happen; I would feel bursts of joy shimmering in my chest; I would take to the malt balls; and within fifteen minutes, I would be miserably full and terribly uncomfortable. I soon realized that whereas I used to eat compulsively when I was sad, angry, or depressed, now I was eating when I was happy. And whereas the expression of sadness, etc., used to be forbidden, joy had now taken its place.

In most circles, it is more acceptable to be miserable than to be happy. It is also safer. No one will be threatened by your suffering, no one will want to take it from you, no one will worry that you have more than she does. No one will hate you for being in pain. You're already as low as it's possible to go, so you don't have to worry about being pushed to the ground.

Tolerating joy means being willing to be happy even though the people around you may be depressed, lonely, or sad. Tolerating joy means being willing to take a chance that someone you care about might be envious or threatened by your happiness. It means becoming aware of the unconscious taboos about joy, the unconscious beliefs about happiness. If misery loves company, for instance, what does happiness love?

Notice what happens this week when you feel a surge of gladness or joy.

What do you say to yourself?

To whom do you express it, and can she/he participate in it with you?

On what assumptions about pain and joy are most of your relationships based?

19. Remember that Thin People Have Cellulite, Get Old, and Die

Many of us, in our fattest thoughts, have wished more than cellulite on those who "just can't gain weight regardless of how many hot fudge sundaes or french fries they eat." This chapter is not about revenge, however. It is about truth.

No matter how thin, gorgeous, rich, and long-legged someone is, she will still have cellulite, get old, and die. And the reason it's important to remember this is because we forget it all the time. We imbue enviable physical and material qualities with a kind of goldenness, as if they confer exemptions from the vicissitudes of being alive. We unconsciously believe that reaching our goals not only gives our lives meaning, but protects us from pain, from cellulite, and from death.

Goals are important, but reaching them does not protect us from anything except the frustration of not reaching them. Grace is not conferred on those who get what everyone else wants. I was starstruck by Jackie Onassis for thirty-one years; I wanted to believe that her mythical life would protect her from illness and pain. When she got cancer, lost her hair, and died, I was finally convinced that there were no exemptions from aging or mortality.

To begin separating the physical goal from the feeling you believe it will confer, make a list of all the things that being thin or achieving your goals has given you.

Be honest. Has it changed the way you feel about your self-worth?

Now, make a list of all the things you thought it would give you that it hasn't.

How can you move toward those things?

What would need to change about your life now so that you could prioritize those things?

What could you do next week?

Tomorrow?

Right now?

20. Eat Enough Fat

Ahh, fat. The dreaded word. I remember hearing Susan Powter shout about it on television one day. "Recognize the word?" she said. "Fat!" Everyone cheered.

"There is a reason it's called fat!"

More cheers.

"Fat makes you fat!"

I'm here to tell you that she is wrong. And she was wrong for two reasons:

1. Since fat is responsible for satiety, when you don't eat enough fat, you never feel full. Which means that you spend your days *grazing*, wandering from Diet Cokes to nonfat chips to salad without dressing to nonfat cake. When you don't eat enough fat, you wonder whether something is wrong with you, why you always feel hungry. You convince yourself that you are bottomless, that you can never get enough.

2. A recent study at the University of California showed that people who were given what they thought was nonfat yogurt ate twice as much as the people given yogurt labeled as containing fat. When we think something doesn't have fat, we fool ourselves into believing it really doesn't count, and we eat more than we usually would. Which means we are getting fat on nonfat foods. Since this latest nonfat craze, Americans have gained an average of eight pounds.

A waiter at an Italian restaurant once complained to me that his customers would be very strict about having their pasta without sauce, their fish without butter, their coffee without cream, and then they would order cannolis and tiramisu for dessert, both of which are made with heavy cream, butter, and sugar.

This is what I have learned about fat:

Too much fat makes you fat.

But *too little* makes you fat, too, because you usually make up for eating nonfat foods by eating twice as much.

I suggest that you speak to a health care professional about your particular situation, about your medical history, about what kinds and amounts of fat are necessary and healthy for you. And then I suggest that you allow yourself to eat enough fat to feel full. Part of the reason that many of us feel as if we could start eating at one end of our kitchens and chomp our way clear across the United States is that we never give ourselves permission to feel full without feeling guilty, to eat enough fat when it's not on a binge.

You really aren't going to devour the universe, but you will never know that until you discover the right balance of fat for your body. Until you allow yourself to eat enough of it to be satisfied.

Repeat after me: Olive oil is not the enemy.

21. Remember that There Is No Right Way, Right Path, Right Answer, Right Food

In every workshop, at least ten people ask me what I think of Overeaters Anonymous, and in every workshop I say the same thing: There is no right way. What works for one person may not work for another. What works at one time in your life may not work five years later. It's important to honor all the paths you've taken, the cures you've tried, the efforts you've made, and to let go of them when they stop assisting your growth.

Be willing to stay current with your life choices.

On a regular basis, ask yourself these five questions about the company you keep, the foods you eat, the work you do, the ways you give and receive love and money.

1. Does it lead you toward a fuller life or does it confine you?

2. Does it bring you closer to your heart or does it take you farther away?

3. Does it open you or does it close you?

4. Does it allow you to trust yourself further or does it make you frightened of yourself?

5. Does it enlarge your life or does it make your life smaller?

If your answer to these questions is consistently on the side of a closed heart, fear, and constriction, it's important to have that information. You can't change what's wrong if you won't even let yourself know it's wrong. The next step, of course, is acting on that awareness without feeling as if you are going to betray your friends or the community with whom you participated in the activity.

Paths are not meant to be followed forever. They are meant to take you from one place to the next. When you use a canoe to cross a river, you don't need to carry the canoe on your back after you've reached land. When a vehicle has served its purpose, it's time to put it down.

2 2 . Wear a Belt

My friend Deborah, who is five feet tall and weighs
ninety pounds, but who once weighed one hundred
forty pounds, says that if she doesn't wear a belt now,
she forgets she has a waist. She forgets she has a body.
She feels like a walking head.

In my experience, most women have no idea what
size their bodies truly are. Ask a friend to show you
how big her stomach is, and she will extend her arms
two feet past her abdomen. Ask a group of women to

show you the size of their thighs, and they will describe hulking mounds with no resemblance to physical anatomy.

Wearing a belt is a simple, concrete way of physically defining yourself. It allows you to circumscribe your body, to actually touch its boundary line. When you wear a belt, you give yourself the chance to distinguish between your ideas about how big you are and your actual body size.

Also, many women have difficulty separating the inside from the outside because there is so much empathy, so much capacity to give nourishment, so much non-physical sensing of another and oneself. In defining your body by a belt, you say: "This is me, this is the exact size of my waist. This is the line I draw between what's inside me and what's outside me. I exist. I am not amorphous."

When you eat a lot or when you binge, wearing a belt can also serve to remind you that you and a small cottage are not the same size.

23. Three Ways to Stop a Fat-and-Ugly Attack

When I teach this material in my workshops, students look at me with blank expressions. Or else they glare at me as if they want to murder me. "But, Geneen," they say, "the attacks are all TRUE! I AM fat. My stomach DOES look like Niagara Falls. How can I stop the attack when what I am attacking myself about is true?"

It doesn't matter what is true and what isn't. What matters is that guilt, shame, blame, and judgment will never lead to change. If they did, the very first diet you went on would have worked forever because diets are built on shame and punishment. If it's true that you are fat, calling yourself a blob of blubber will not lead to losing weight, although it will probably lead you straight to the refrigerator. If it's true that you lied to a friend, shaming yourself until you feel like a whimpering cockroach will not help you discover why you were afraid to tell the truth.

To change what you do, you have to be able to think.

To think, you have to stop the attack.

To stop the attack, here are three things you can do:

1. Go outside where no one can hear you. As loud as you can, say "SHUT UP!" Feel free to curse, especially if you never use the "f" word. You need to shock this part of you into leaving you alone. You need to talk to this voice the way you would have talked to your parents if you had no respect for them, if you didn't care whether they loved you or not, if you were convinced that they were trying to take away every last shred of happiness you had.

2. Drop the rope. End the tug-of-war. Agree with the content of the attack. "You're right. I am selfish, controlling, and look like a tub of lard, but what can I do? I was born that way." During a particularly heated fight with Matt recently, he grabbed a raw egg and cracked it on his own head. The fight instantly ended in astonishment and giggles; it's impossible to stay angry with someone who has yolk dripping on his face.

3. Recognize the attack for what it is. As soon as you understand what's going on, you are no longer caught. You no longer believe that the TRUTH is being spoken. At this point, you can brush it off. "Oh, there you go again, saying the same old thing." Or you can treat it with humor. "You think I'm eating a lot now? You should have seen what I ate for breakfast!" Or, you can firmly say, "You are not my friend." Which is true.

The important thing is to disengage from the viciousness of the attack. Most people get caught because they are so used to speaking to themselves this way, they don't even know that an attack has taken place. Every time you use the words "should," "shouldn't," "right," or "wrong," you are probably attacking yourself.

Remember that change can only come from understanding and the action you take from that understanding. The greatest single block to change is the hypnotic power this voice has over you. Every time you defend yourself against an attack, you develop the strength, power, and courage to truly change.

24. When There Are Tigers Above You and Tigers Below You, Eat a Ripe Strawberry

ꙩ

This is my version of an ancient Buddhist story.

A woman was jogging in the forest when she realized that a family of tigers had leaped from a mountain and was momentarily going to be feasting on her for their next meal. She started to run very fast. After years of aerobics classes, years of weight training, and two months of the newest exercise—spinning—she could outrace even the famed physically fit tiger. But alas, since she had been running on treadmills and not in forests, she wasn't used to navigating her way through dense trees, and ran right up to the edge of a cliff. Ever resourceful, she scampered down the side and hung on to a clump of vines.

Meanwhile, the tigers gathered above her, breathing heavily and licking their lips with their huge, rough tongues. Then she heard a roaring below her and saw another family of tigers making their way up the cliff. Apparently, this second family also intended to use her as dinner, and they were fast approaching. "Lean as my body is," she thought (and smiled for the briefest millisecond as she remembered her last under-water fat test—only 18 percent body fat), "it is probably Zone favorable and will make a fine dinner for these beasts."

Just then she heard a faint rustle and saw a small field mouse chomping through the vines to which she clung. "It's curtains for me," she said to the mouse. "All this work at being thin and look where it got me." At that moment, she noticed a ripe strawberry hanging from the vine. Since she had been on a high-protein diet that forbade fruit of any kind, she hadn't tasted a strawberry in a long, long time.

With tigers above, and tigers below, her life flashed before her: the years she had spent running away from the past and toward an imagined, better future, believing that true love and joy were waiting right around the corner. All those ripe-strawberry moments she had passed up, waiting for riper strawberries, for better moments, for her life really, truly to begin. Surrounded by tigers, she realized there was only one thing to do: eat the ripe strawberry. And although she did not live happily ever after, she enjoyed that strawberry more than she'd enjoyed anything, ever.

There are always tigers above us and tigers below us, and even so, we refuse to eat that juicy, ripe strawberry hanging an inch away.

Again and again I've heard the same story: A student of mine loses weight, arrives at the moment she has been waiting for, but then her mother gets ill or her child breaks his arm or her husband loses his job. She escapes the tigers of food and weight, runs smack into the tigers of ill health and lost jobs, and forgets to enjoy the strawberries on the way.

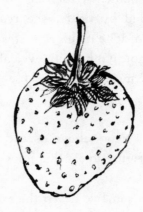

We have no choice about the tigers above and the tigers below. Pain is a part of life. You manage to get one part under control and another part falls apart. You may be lucky enough to experience an oasis of time in which everything is smooth, everyone is well, and you are also thin. Whether it lasts an hour, a week, a month, a year, eventually there will be more tigers. But there will also be more strawberries. The sun will keep coming up, your child will say something that will crack your heart open, a new friend will appear, and you will once again be struck by the unbearable wonder and tenderness of life.

Most of us ignore the strawberries because we believe that there's something even better up ahead. We spend our youth waiting for our lives to begin, we get old waiting for our lives to begin, and we die waiting for our lives to begin. As if there were such a thing as finally getting it all right. As if perfection really exists.

A certain kind of perfection does exist, even though the tigers will never go away. Perfection is choosing to enjoy the lusciousness life offers in whatever form it presents itself, even when you are not as thin as you want to be, you owe money to the IRS, and someone you love is dying.

When there are tigers above you and tigers below you, there will always be a strawberry right in front of you. Pick it. Enjoy it. Let yourself have that much.

25. Stare at Normal Women's Bodies (Normal Does Not Include Models, Actresses, and Elite Athletes)

Every summer for four or five days, I go to a Zen retreat center in Carmel Valley and stare at naked women's bodies. Some would call this peeping. I call it observing spiritual reality. Because as I sit in the women's baths, soaking in the mineral springs and swimming in the stream, this is what I see: sagging breasts, dimpled buttocks, cellulite thighs, stretch marks, flabby stomachs, and drooping underarms. Oh yes, I did see one body that looked like the glossy ideal. On a ten-year-old.

When I look at bodies of normal women, I am reminded that no one looks like the pictures we see in magazines. Even the models don't look like the pictures we see of them. Photographs are often retouched to erase a few inches from the legs and the arms, and remove any cellulite, sags, droops, or imperfections that make a body human.

A few years ago, when my picture was taken for the cover of my book *Appetites*, I had a mole on my forehead. I asked the art director at the publishing company to remove it from the photograph, and with one magical stroke of the computer, it was gone. Giddy from the power of being able to alter my face so easily, I thought, "Gee, what would it be like if he removed some of those wrinkles around my eyes and took away just an eensy, teensy part of the fullness of my face?" I was getting giddier by the moment, thinking of how gorgeous I could look with my eyes a little larger, my cheeks a little thinner, my hair a little thicker. When I spoke to the art director about making more changes, he said, "But, Geneen, then you won't look like yourself."

I felt like saying, "Oh that..." when I remembered that *Appetites* was about self-acceptance, and the desire to change my face was possibly maybe perhaps a bit hypocritical.

Normal women have wrinkles, sags, and cellulite. But since we don't compare ourselves to normal women, we end up feeling as if our bodies are wrong. As if our imperfect bodies are an indication that we are not working hard enough, don't care passionately enough, have let ourselves go. When we compare ourselves to airbrushed, computerized bodies, we believe that if we drank enough water, ate the right combinations of food, and exercised the requisite thirty minutes four days a week, we could look like that, too.

Drinking enough water, eating nourishing food, and exercising a few times a week are all loving ways to treat our bodies. But if we engage in those activities with the hope that they will make us look like airbrushed photographs or prepubescent girls, we will live in a perpetual state of disappointment and self-loathing.

Take a good, long stare at real women's bodies in the mall or grocery store. So they have wrinkles or cellulite or sags. So what. That is what living looks like. That is what loving and losing and hoping and caring does to bodies. The goal of life is not to get through to the end and wind up looking like you just began.

After you've looked at normal women's bodies, look at yourself in the mirror. Stand there for at least three minutes, once a week, for six weeks. Every time you notice a stretch mark, a sag, a wrinkle, say to yourself, "This is what living looks like. This is what loving looks like." And you will be telling the truth.

26. Wear Your Special-Occasion Clothes Any Old Day

Sometimes it is necessary to wear gold sequins to go to the corner store. Sometimes at 8 A.M. when you take your child to school you need to wear a black velvet top that flutters like a butterfly. There is no good reason to save your special-occasion clothes for special occasions. Think of all the pleasure you miss if you do.

The times when I believe it is absolutely necessary to wear your dishy, gorgeous clothes are after a binge or on a particularly fat, ugly, or miserable day when you tend to gravitate toward the stained, ragged, baggy sweatpants that could fit you and three other people. These are the times when you need to remind yourself that there is someone home who is not a shapeless, oozing banana slug.

Other days—any old days—are still worthy of your best clothes. What's the point of saving what you love most for two or three times a year? Why not wear velvet to buy a carton of milk? Why not flutter around the grocery store feeling resplendent? I know this may sound excessive or silly, but what's silly about feeling gorgeous every single day?

Last week, three of Matt's female cousins visited us from New York. After dinner, the conversation drifted in the direction of shopping and clothes, a subject on which I am well versed, and I began to expound on my theory of wearing special-occasion clothes on any old day. They looked at me, aghast. What about grape juice stains? Coffee spills? I asked if they could remember the last time they drank grape juice. (The answer was no.) I reminded them of napkins. "Spills happen," I said. "What's the point of keeping unspilledupon clothes in your closet, waiting for the time you finally feel special enough to wear them? What about taking the bull by the horns?" (I was beginning to get a little carried away). "What about using your clothes to *initiate* the inner sense of feeling thin, gorgeous, and happy, rather than waiting until you feel those things to wear them?"

"Show us what you wear to the grocery store," they said. I took them downstairs and showed them my black velvet top that looks like a butterfly. Then I showed them my shimmery green top that looks like a dewy forest morning. Soon, the floor and chairs were heaped with clothes and they were parading in front of the mirror in diaphanous jackets and flowing pants, trying to imagine themselves doing errands in such unerrand-like clothes. They giggled. They felt as if someone had just given them permission to eat ice cream for breakfast. They realized they were slaves of fashion etiquette and that it was better to wear a favorite shirt and spill something on it than never to wear it at all.

I know there are days when it's either impractical to wear an off-the-shoulder sheath or you just don't feel like looking like a butterfly or a forest. Most of the time when I write, I wear the same gaudy red, purple, and yellow flowered leggings. I want to be comfortable, and soft, old clothes make me feel that way. But there are also days when I wake up feeling lost and disoriented and my whole life seems wrong. Or days when I just want to feel beautiful, even if I am staying home the whole day or only going out for a carton of milk. On these days, I put on a beautiful shirt, a colorful sweater — some article of clothing that will evoke an inner recognition that light and beauty and expansion are right here, right now.

The important thing is not to replace one set of "should's" with another. There is nothing you should or should not wear to the store. There are no rules.

You get to decide what goes in your body and on it.

Wearing special-occasion clothes on any old day means being willing to believe that you are special on every old (and new!) day. It means expanding your definition of lusciousness—and thereby relieving food of the need to be everything, all kinds of sweetness and pleasure. It means giving yourself permission to wear scrumptious things as well as to touch, taste, and eat them.

27. More About Presence: The Practice of Sensing Your Arms and Legs

When I talk about presence in my workshops, students give me suspicious stares. Some of them decide they don't like me or want their money back. Presence sounds dumb. "C'mon, Geneen. You make it sound so simple. What about my lousy relationship or the fact that I have three kids under the age of five and not one second for myself the entire day? How can I 'be with my life as it is,' if that life makes me unhappy?" Good question, I say. And it is.

In the beginning, practicing presence needs to stay very simple, which is to say that presence is not sexy, is not glamorous, is not exciting or dramatic. In the beginning, presence is not about changing relationships or going to therapy or making yourself crazy in the middle of a hectic day by having to go off somewhere and Show Up. You start exactly where you are, with all the ingredients and distractions in your life that drive you crazy. When you practice presence, you learn to be with those things in an entirely different and spacious way.

The main practice of presence is to sense your arms and legs. Another way of saying this is that you become *embodied*. The reason this is helpful is because your thoughts can drive you insane. There is no particular pattern to them; in a split second, they zing crazily from the time you fell from your swing when you were five to what you are going to say to the person who insulted you yesterday. If you try to follow your thoughts, you get lost in fantasies, resentments, anticipated disappointments. There is no ground beneath you, nothing solid to hold on to, no way of bringing yourself back to what you are doing now, this very second. You get to the end of a day—or the end of your life—and you wonder where you've been. And the answer is, Lost in thought!

You are already in your body, but you hardly ever realize it because you get so lost in thinking about the past and the future. Since your arms and legs are with you now, they are a perfect place to land. Also, they are not usually a place that is filled with emotion (like your heart or your throat or even your eyes), which makes them a fine place to place your awareness.

In the mornings, before you get out of bed, begin sensing (i.e., focusing your attention and paying attention to the sensations that arise) your right foot—the toes, the ankle, the back of your foot, the arch. Then, as if you were squeezing a tube of toothpaste, move your attention up through your calf, your shin, your knee. Continue moving your awareness all the way up through the right hip, and then the right hand, the fingers, the wrist, the elbow. When you get to the shoulder, move across to your left shoulder and down this arm to the hand, and from the left hip to the left foot. This should take about five minutes.

During the day, every time you remember, sense your arms and legs again. Just for a few seconds. (I do this about a hundred times a day.) This will help you land in your body, bring your mind back to the present moment, give you a kind of mountain-solid feeling.

When you are present, nothing is missing. Time seems to stretch. And the reason it does is because it is our thoughts, our crowded, worried minds that make us feel so rushed. When you are present, a day seems like a week, a month like a year.

Presence enables you to see that this body, your home, the place you've spent years trying to change, is a pretty cool place to be.

28. No Matter What You've Consumed in the Past Twenty-four Hours, Twenty-four Days, or Twenty-four Years, Eat the Very Next Time You Get Hungry

During my dieting heydays, I made one agreement with myself again and again: "Okay," I would say, "you can eat this cake, but tomorrow, you have to fast." Then I would finish the entire cake, trying to store up for the hunger to come. When tomorrow came, I would feel miserable, irritable, and deprived. I would starve myself for a day, maybe two, after which I would feel either self-righteous or crazed from being so hungry. Either way, I would take a headlong dive into food, overeat once more, and convince myself that I could not be trusted around food. My hunger was my enemy. I was certain I wanted too much of everything — food, love, comfort.

In my classes, I call this "messing around with your hunger." It's like trying to get the right temperature in your house by turning the thermostat all the way up, then ratcheting it all the way down, then up again, then down again, and doing this all day long for ten years. After a while, the self-regulatory mechanism breaks from being messed with too much, and you start to think something is wrong with the thermostat.

If you don't trust your hunger, it's because you've messed with it too much for too long.

Starving yourself after overeating only leads to another cycle of overeating and starving yourself. It doesn't lead to weight loss, health, well-being, or balanced energy. It also makes you feel like a lunatic, since hunger is a survival mechanism. You need to eat to live. When you deny your hunger, even the day after you've consumed thousands of calories, you are also denying the life force that keeps you alive.

Eating when you are hungry is *not* what causes

you to gain weight. When you eat from body hunger, you develop trust and confidence in your ability to care for yourself. Eating when you are hungry allows you to relax. Think of a hungry, crying infant. Her body gets red, tight, rigid, anxious when she needs food. As soon as the hunger is satisfied, she relaxes. Her jangled nervous system becomes fluid again. Everything is right with the world.

Hunger is basic, primal, enlivening. Years of dieting or deprivation or judging our bodies have made us forget that hunger is actually the signal that informs us it's time to eat. We are so used to eating because it's in front of us, eating because everyone else is eating, eating to celebrate, eating to commiserate that we've forgotten that hunger is natural, instinctive, and ultimately trustworthy. After a lifetime of messing around with it, it's possible that you've forgotten how to respond to your own hunger. It's possible that you no longer hear or trust its signals. We've become so brainwashed by every food fad (pasta is good; pasta is bad; oat bran is good; oat bran is bad; milk is a good source of calcium for your bones; milk leaches calcium from your bones; the Zone is the answer; forget the Zone — food combining will save you) that we've forgotten how to listen to what we truly need.

It's time to start over. Starving yourself will never, ever lead to permanent weight loss. More important, it will always lead to a ragged, empty feeling of desperation. If you can't listen to and trust one of the most basic drives you have, you begin to feel that there is no ground to stand on. No way of knowing what you need, no trust in your ability to get it.

No matter what you have eaten, no matter how fat or ugly you feel, it is crucial that you begin listening to your hunger now, today. You don't need to eat for "the hunger to come." The next time you get hungry, you can eat again.

Practice listening to your hunger/fullness signals when you are and aren't hungry by closing your eyes for thirty seconds a few times a day, becoming aware of three different areas: your mouth, your heart, and your stomach. Ask yourself, "If these areas could talk to me about hunger, what would they say? Do they want food? Do they want something else? Contact?

Quiet attention?" Then, rate your physical hunger on a scale of one to ten. One is very hungry, five is comfortable, ten is stuffed. If you are at four or below, you are hungry. Also rate your emotional hunger. One is empty, five is fine, and ten is feeling great. If you are physically hungry, think about what you want to eat, what would feel good in your body, and eat it. If you are emotionally hungry (heart or mouth hunger), consider what would nourish you. Remember that no matter how sad or lonely or angry you feel, eating will not take it away. If you eat when you are not hungry, all that will happen is that you will still be sad or lonely or angry, and also full.

When you are physically hungry, eat. When you are physically hungry, nothing but food will satisfy you. I will tell you what I tell my students: You need to develop a voice inside that says, "It's okay, honey. You don't have to be afraid of yourself any longer. Trust your hungers. Rest when you are tired, ask for love when you need it, and eat when you are hungry." Amen.

29. ...And Stop When You've Had Enough

෨Ꭷ

Ah-ha," you are saying to yourself, "I knew there was a catch!" And you're right, there is.

It's about what you hear when you hear the word "enough."

It's about what you believe you can't get enough of.

It's about taking more than enough of something you know you can get — food — because you believe it's impossible to get enough of what you really, really want. Love. Joy. Value. Happiness. Money. Contentment. Success. Sex. Understanding. Friendship.

This much is certain: Five or ten dollars will buy you *a lot* of food. With five or ten dollars in your pocket, you can get more than enough to eat.

Food is not the problem.

When I first started doing this work, people would say to me, "I can't believe you're saying I can eat what I want. You don't know *me*. If I ate what I wanted, I'd eat three dozen doughnuts, a gallon of ice cream, and a pizza — and that would be the appetizer. Not dieting might work for other people, but it wouldn't work for me."

The unspoken message was, I want everything, and I'll never stop wanting everything. There is not enough food in the world to fill this hunger. I will never be full enough.

After throwing copies of my books against the wall a few dozen times, telling me I was crazy, and rebelling against what I was saying by going on yet another diet, which was followed by another binge, they would eventually come back and say, "You might be crazy, but I'm desperate and nothing else seems to work, so now what?"

These are the now whats:

ﾟ The easiest place to begin learning about enough is where you are living right now: your body. When you learn that you can get enough food, that you can actually be satisfied with much less than you imagine, you will begin to trust that you are not bottomless, that you will not be forever hungry. You will develop confidence, not just in your ability to have enough food, but in the possibility of having whatever you believe you can't get enough of.

ﾟ If you start eating when you are not physically hungry, it is very difficult to stop when you've had enough. It is like pouring water into an already full glass. There's no space for the food to fill.

ﾟ Being full and having enough are not necessarily the same thing. You can have enough without being full.

❧ You are allowed to have enough when there is still food left on your plate. The starving children in Bangladesh will not benefit from your leftovers.

❧ Having enough food is both physical and emotional. If you don't eat what you want, if you are not present while you are eating, if you miss the entire eating experience by either talking or watching television or getting lost in fantasy, you will finish the meal and feel as if you didn't get enough. Satisfaction depends on being present. If there is no one home inside your body to receive the nourishment, no one can register the signal of enough.

❧ You can stop eating when you've physically had enough even though you haven't yet figured out how to fill the nonfood-related hungers. Simply being aware of the difference between physical and emotional hunger, and knowing that all the food in the world will not fill hunger that is not physical, allows you to decide to stop eating when you've had enough. The rest will follow.

꙰ When you stop using food to feed the hungers of your heart, you open a door to secrets you've been keeping from yourself. To quiet needs. To unspoken desires. To what would satisfy you deeply. You begin to discover the subtleties of what makes you you: "Oh, I see. It's not food I want, I'm just tired, and I need to rest." Or "Oh, I get it. I think taking time by myself is indulgent, so I eat and give myself some space that way."

Stopping when you've had enough food will lead to naming what you truly want. Instead of living your life crowded onto one note—food—you become a warm, rich chord, a whole symphony.

30. Remind Yourself That It's Already Broken

At a meditation retreat I attended in 1982, the teacher held up his favorite teacup and said, "As far as I'm concerned, this cup is already broken." My back was killing me from spending fifteen hours a day sitting cross-legged on a cushion, waking up at four-thirty in the morning, and eating gruel for breakfast. I was very cranky. When he said that, my first thought was, "Huh?" and my second thought was, "Oh, for God's sake, stop talking gibberish and ring the bell so I can go eat some trail mix."

Since then, I've given some thought to the concept of "it's already broken," and I think that teacher may have been on to something.

When I got my first new car a few years ago, my husband, Matt, bumped into four cement walls within five days, leaving huge gashes in the front fender. I was furious. I accused him of the worst sin — being a New Yorker who drove like a Californian. And then I remembered it was already scratched, it was already broken. I decided to stay married after all.

The nature of things is that if they don't get lost, they get stolen, and if they don't get stolen, they get broken, and if they don't get broken, they fade or fall apart. This law applies to teacups, cars, people, sweaters, pets, computers, earrings, and just about everything you can touch or buy or have.

How does it help to know that, although "it" is in one piece now, its eventual, inevitable state is "already broken"?

It helps you fully appreciate what you've got while you have it. Instead of protecting it, being worried about losing it, or spending your time and energy devising ways to keep it safe forever, you place your at-

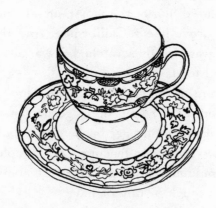

tention and love right square in this moment, and you luxuriate in every last bit of it. Whether it's the perfect sweater, the most beautiful vase, a magnificent sunset, the deliciously romantic phase of a new relationship, or a new car, knowing that it won't last forever can help you be wildly appreciative of it now.

And lest you begin wallowing in the anticipated sadness of losing a particular form, consider what my mother told me when I was fifteen and someone else bought the leopard-print headband at Campus Corner because I waited too long to go back for it: "There's always more where that came from, darling."

31. Lagniappe

Lagniappe (pronounced LAN-yap) is an expression I learned when I lived in New Orleans. It means a beneficent kind of extra, an extra you weren't expecting, but are now immensely glad to have.

When you understand that "it's already broken," your whole life becomes lagniappe.

You know those stories about people who come back from near-death experiences forever changed? Forever grateful to just be alive? And those stories about dying people with cancer who say that cancer is a gift? That they wouldn't change places with anyone in the world?

These people all seem to know the same thing: how to celebrate being alive. They take nothing for granted because they've faced their own brokenness, and know that eventually everything, including themselves, will be broken again.

The same thing happens on a much smaller scale when you lose a precious possession and then find it again. Suddenly, you are extravagantly happy—happier than you were before you lost it. When you lose what you love, it makes you realize its preciousness; when you find it again, you are given a second chance to celebrate what was always there. You already lost it, and now, every second you have with it is precious.

The value of understanding the meaning of lagniappe is living the rest of your life as if you've just found your lost wallet.

A man who was dying of AIDS, said, "I've grown to love this way of life—the intensity, the clarity, the poignancy. The ability to see things at their value, to measure life, at last, by its true and terminal standard. I laugh louder these days and cry at nothing. I work until my fingers hurt and I exercise my heart in love. The future is a fantasy and I think almost nothing about the past."

When you face the inevitable — that people, as well as possessions, get broken — and when you live as if you and they already are — every single, blessed thing you see, feel, and touch is lagniappe.

3 2. Develop Friendships That Applaud Your Strengths and Celebrate Your Successes

A friend is not a friend when she doesn't want the best for you. A friend is not a friend when she is envious of your happiness. A friend is not a friend when you find yourself keeping secrets from her because you fear that if you told the truth, she would be hurt or lonely or unhappy with her own life. A friend is not a friend if there is no room for expansion, joy, happiness, change. If she does not want you to be the best you can be, to have all you can possibly have, to be as successful and as gorgeous as you have the potential to be, she is not your friend.

When my parents got divorced, my mother lost almost all her friends. It was okay with them when she was unhappy in her marriage, it was okay with them when she had affairs with other men; most of them were unhappy and having affairs as well. But when my mother had the courage to change her life by getting divorced, even her best friend, the one she talked to every day, cut off all contact with her.

Friends often have unspoken rules about what is allowed and what is forbidden. Some of these rules may be: You have to stay equally miserable; you have to stay equally fat; you can't move to another city, change jobs, change relationships, or begin working at something that takes you away from each other.

When you begin snipping off your happiness to match the size of your friend's unhappiness, it is time to take a serious look at the friendship. It's important that you be kind to yourself and to your friend as you do this. It's important that you continue to value all that you have shared and still share: the goodness, the love, the things you have in common. It is rarely a black-or-white situation; if it were, you probably would have left a long time ago.

Not every friendship is meant to last forever. Some friendships are meant to lead you to other friendships. Some are meant to be short, intense experiences. Some are meant to teach you one particular thing. And some, of course, are meant to be lifelong.

It takes courage, maturity, honesty, and a reservoir of self-love to assess the vitality of a friendship.

Make it a priority to develop friendships that applaud your strengths and celebrate your successes. You are worth being truly loved and supported, and there are people you haven't met, friends you haven't made who would do a fabulous job at both.

33. ... And Begin to Gently Let Go of Friends Who Don't Want the Best for You

~

This year, my relationship with a close friend ended. When we met fifteen years ago, we shared the same values, used the same language to describe our feelings, were drawn to the same people. But, slowly over the past eight years, our ideas of support and being our best selves changed in ways we never anticipated, and we could not find a common meeting ground. Though we tried everything we knew to do, our interactions became agonizing.

If people had told me five years ago that this friend would not be in my life today, I would have told them that we adored each other and were committed to working through any difficulties. I would have told them they were crazy. "Friendships are to be cherished," I would have said, "especially long-time friends." And while I still believe that, I no longer believe that you should cherish them at any cost. When it is consistently more painful to have a friend in your life than not, it is time to let go of the relationship.

How do you do this?

You begin by telling yourself the truth. "Every time I tell her something good, she changes the subject." Or, "I feel as if something is wrong with me when I am around her." Or, "I'd better not share this with her, it will make her feel bad."

You say this truth out loud, either to someone you trust or to your journal. You get it out of your head and into the world.

You imagine what your life would be like without this person. The parts that would be better, the parts that would be worse. You imagine not having to pretend or hide or diminish yourself when you are with this person. You also imagine the loneliness you would feel without this person in your life.

You feel what your relationship is really like with this friend. You stop trying to protect yourself from the pain, both of losing her, and of losing yourself when you are with her.

If it's possible, you share these feelings with your friend. She might hear you, she might want to change. She might be grateful for the feedback. And she might not.

If she can hear what you say, you work together to create a different kind of relationship. It's worth the effort.

If she can't hear you without criticizing you or getting defensive, the limitations of this friendship will become apparent.

You may decide that the joys of this friendship far outweigh its limitations. And you may not.

If you allow yourself to be fully aware of the truth, and if the truth is that this friendship is more painful than supportive, it will eventually lose its attraction. There will be no energy between the two of you. Ideally, if you allow what's already there to unfold and don't protect yourself from the truth, the passage will be smooth. But it might be painful. You might have to grieve. After a while, letting go will seem easier than holding on, and at that point, separation will then be an act of love for both of you.

Note: Ending a friendship does not mean that you're blaming someone else for your pain or closing your heart to your friend. Neither does it discount the possibility that the two of you might again be friends. Ending a friendship means that you acknowledge that this relationship is creating more ill-will than love, more pain than joy, and is therefore not serving the best interests of either of you *at this time*.

34. Eliminate the Ways You Gain Weight Without Eating

We all have ways we manage to get food into our mouths without counting what we do as eating.

This is my friend Cory's list:

1. rearranging broken cookies

2. when someone else is paying

3. anything with a diet soda

4. cleaning off the kids' plates

5. when I'm cooking

6. driving in the car

7. any food I don't like

8. when it's for medicinal purposes

9. before exercise

10. after exercise

11. during sex

12. when my mother-in-law comes to visit

13. if it's eaten frozen and it's not meant to be

To this, I would add the time-honored tradition of "edging a cake": taking off a little on each side so that the next person who comes along won't be disturbed by the asymmetry. When you eat an edge here and an edge there, it doesn't really count as cake. It counts as altruism.

Make your own list of the ways you eat and gain weight without counting what you do as eating. The purpose of making this list is simply to become more conscious. Also, to give yourself permission to actually enjoy what you eat. If you are going to eat cake anyway, why not enjoy it? Why not cut yourself a piece, make noises while you eat, and taste every last drop of butter, flour, and sugar?

After you've made your list, pat yourself on the back. It takes ingenuity to come up with some of these methods. Give yourself some credit. And then give yourself permission to do openly what you are going to do anyway. If you are going to eat thirteen pieces of a broken cookie, eat a whole one instead. Savor it. Then move on to the rest of your day.

Now, decide which ingenious ways are the easiest to stop, and then one by one, one each week, stop doing them.

35. When Things Begin to Fall Apart, Let Them

Uh-oh. You were following me until now. You were nodding your head, saying, "Yeah, I can do that, yeah, that sounds good," but this is going too far. So I'll tell you a story.

At a workshop a few months ago, I worked with a woman whose husband had died a year and a half before. They'd been married for twenty years and, in her words, "adored each other." Now she woke up alone each day and she ate. And ate. Since his death, she had gained fifty pounds, with no end in sight. "I can feel my waist expanding as we speak," she said.

"You must be so sad," I offered.

She nodded. "But most of the time, instead of feeling the grief, I eat."

"What would happen if you let yourself feel it?"

"I'd fall apart," she said.

"And then what?" I asked.

"There is no 'then what' in there. I'd be a mess. I'd go insane. "

"Can you let yourself feel the grief for five minutes right now?"

She nodded her head. "It's never very far." And then she cried, and two hundred of us cried with her. Four minutes later, she stopped crying. I asked her what had happened.

"It's over for now. But it felt very good to just let myself feel sad." She looked around. "Nothing happened. My body didn't disintegrate. I didn't go crazy."

"What would happen if you let yourself feel it in five-minute increments at home?"

She was silent for a long time. "I'm frightened," she finally said, "that I would eventually feel happy, and then I would betray my husband. It would be as if he weren't ever alive. At least this way, I still have his memory and I also have food. Gaining weight makes me feel so unattractive that I don't even consider the possibility of dating again."

"So being happy is a betrayal of the love you and he shared?"

A grin slowly appeared on her face, and then she started to laugh. "Gee, when you say it out loud, I realize how convoluted that really is. He would want me to be happy. He *loved* me." The whole room began to clap. She beamed and sat down.

The moral of the story is, If you don't let yourself fall apart when everything in you *has already* fallen apart, you will sleepwalk through your life, you will live in limbo. You will eat to numb the pain, then thread your feelings through the layers of weight you gain. You will eat. You will not stop eating.

Just as we have an entire set of beliefs about happiness, we also have a set about pain. And the most common one is that if we let ourselves feel it, we will be overwhelmed, go insane, fall apart, be unable to function, turn into blobby messes. But that is a child's view of pain, not an adult's view. Nothing lasts forever, including pain. For some reason, we believe that if we speak about our happiness it will disappear, but that pain will last forever.

This is the thing: What you don't let begin can never end.

And this is the second thing: If you don't let yourself fall apart, you will never be completely together.

So, the next time you feel as if you are falling apart:

ꙮ Set a timer.

ꙮ Cry as hard as you can for five minutes.

ꙮ When the timer rings, get up.

ꙮ Go on with your day. Wash the dishes. Pick up your child at school.

The next time you are falling apart, set your timer for five minutes, find a soft place, and fall.

36. Ask for Help:
You Can't Do It Alone

We need help. It's that simple. We live in a culture that encourages change by using deprivation and shame. Anorexically thin women are the standard of beauty. Quiet self-reflection is considered self-indulgent or lazy. And the answer is always in something you don't have, don't know, or need to buy. The language of curiosity, kindness, and acting on your own behalf is foreign where we live; it is like speaking Serbo-Croatian in Chinatown.

When a tree is tender and young, first making its roots, a gardener knows to fence it from deer, fertilize it with nutrients, pay loving attention as it gets started. The gardener doesn't grow the tree; she provides the conditions in which it can thrive. We need to do the same with our souls, hearts, spirits, bodies. We need to provide the conditions in which we can thrive, and those conditions involve other people. We need to put ourselves in circumstances in which we can be seen, heard, and loved for who we are and want to become.

We are so used to battering ourselves around. To toughing it out. To taking care of everyone else and not looking after ourselves. We are used to throwing the seeds of our lives in soil and not paying them one more minute of attention. In fact, we do the opposite. We stamp on our hearts. We attack and punish ourselves. We don't trust our fundamental desire to move toward the light, especially when it comes to food, dieting, and weight. The personal and cultural pull is to believe that everything would be all right if we could just shut our mouths or eat just grapefruit or cabbage soup for two weeks.

In every workshop I teach, we form support groups that meet weekly for two to three hours. They are leaderless groups that are based on the principles of curiosity, kindness, and acting on your own behalf— with food and in life. But you don't have to attend a Breaking Free® workshop to be in a support group, nor do you need to be in a support group to ask for help. Groups are simply convenient, structured, prearranged times in which support is available. You can find people of like mind and heart right now, right where you live. They don't have to be your best friends.

Think about what you need. What are the parts of yourself that need loving attention, watering, protection? Think about how you can attend to those needs. Does a group sound appealing to you? If so, put an ad in a weekly paper. That's how I got started. I put an ad in the Santa Cruz *Good Times* paper saying that I wanted to start a group for women who wished to deal with their difficulties with food but without dieting. Ten women called. We decided on a day of the week, time, and place, and I started developing exercises we could do together. Since then, I've written

Why Weight, a book of exercises especially designed for leaderless support groups.

If you are not "a group person," there are many other ways to receive support so that you don't sink back into familiar, unkind patterns. Meet weekly with someone at your church or temple. Join a reading group. Find a counselor, therapist, or spiritual adviser.

The support of which I am speaking is for your whole being. For everything you want to become. For telling the truth. For being spacious with yourself and others. Support for your heart's desires, for what you value most about being alive. My experience is that once you understand the need for this kind of help and open yourself to it—by asking around, by going to events at which you might meet people of like mind, by meditating, by praying—you begin to find it. And once you begin to experience it, you realize you are part of a community of people who want to live with the very same kind of openness, love, curiosity, joy, and humor toward themselves and all beings as you do.

In her poem, "The Low Road," Marge Piercy writes:

Two people can keep each other
sane, can give support, conviction,
love, massage, hope, sex.
Three people are a delegation,
a committee, a wedge. With four
you can play bridge and start
an organization. With six
you can rent a whole house,
eat pie for dinner with no
seconds, and hold a fund raising party.
A dozen make a demonstration.
A hundred fill a hall.
A thousand have solidarity and your own newsletter;
ten thousand, power and your own paper;
a hundred thousand, your own media;
ten million, your own country.

The difference between asking for and receiving help is like the difference between trying to hold yourself up in midair and floating in a swimming pool. The first requires unbelievable effort and is still impossible. The second is a natural function of being supported by the environment in which you place yourself. When you ask for help, hurdles of the mind and heart that seemed totally insurmountable on your own become effortless. Anything is possible.

Except the part about not having enough pie for seconds. That's unacceptable.

37. When You Are Not Hungry, Beauty Is Better than Bonbons

Sometimes, all it takes to remind us that life is infinitely spacious, luscious, and forgiving is resting your eyes on something beautiful. The sun splashing through the dining room at four in the afternoon. Your grandmother's lace tablecloth. A hundred-year-old oak tree. A seashell. A piece of turquoise. A single pale pink peony.

A friend of mine is teaching a course on beauty. She says that we put so much emphasis on function and efficiency that we forget to surround ourselves with beauty. She says that beauty relaxes our soul because, like a poem, its unique purpose is simply to be. For the joy of it. For the expression of it. Just because.

Beauty does not further us along in our careers, help us to relate, instruct us on how to be kind or successful or thin. In our time-crunched, self-important, goal-oriented world, beauty reminds us that not everything can, or should be, measured, weighed, or written down in our date books.

We have the capacity to feel expansive and open and shimmery, not because we have met our goals for the month or because we have accomplished something big, but just because we are alive. Beauty reminds us of that capacity.

When you're hungry, but not for something to eat, take a "beautiful break." The effort itself will prompt you to really *look*, to bathe your eyes in it. Don't stint. Don't be ashamed. Beauty nourishes, it fills. Light a gardenia candle. Gaze at the sky. Rediscover the painting you bought three years ago, and have not truly looked at since.

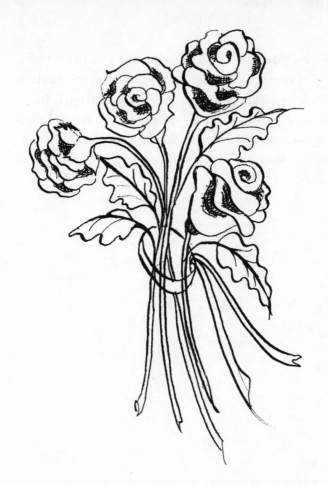

When you're not hungry, beauty is better than a piece of cheesecake. Better than mashed potatoes. Better than a hamburger and milkshake and french fries.

Beauty is fluffy, buttery, creamy, silky, rich, exquisitely sweet, whole-body food. It feeds your eyes, ears, heart, skin, soul all at once. And it doesn't have any calories.

38. Practice Saying No

To parties you don't want to go to, to sex you don't
want to have, to people you don't want to be with, to
activities that drain your energy. To the phone ringing
when you don't want to pick it up. To the ways you
sell your soul.

All too often women say yes with their voices, but
no with their bodies. We allow our weight to speak for
us: Sorry, I can't go to that party, I feel too fat. Sorry,
I can't go to that wedding, I don't fit into any of my

clothes. Sorry, I can't go on that vacation, I wouldn't dare try on bathing suits now. Sorry, I can't be in a relationship right now, no one would be attracted to me. Sorry, I can't have sex with you, I don't want you to see my body with the lights on. Don't want you to touch my stomach. Don't want to be touched at all.

We use food and extra body weight as an excuse to be still, be quiet, be left alone. Since many of us believe that, regardless of what we get paid to do, our real jobs are to be on call for people who need us, we leave ourselves with one way to get what we need and want: food. And since extra body weight also makes us miserable, we never allow ourselves to bask in the luxury of actually having what we want, what we need. There is always a price to saying no with your body, and the price is feeling terrible about yourself.

A friend's therapist told her, "Every time you say yes when you mean no, you abandon yourself. And every time you say no when you mean no, you create a place inside from which you can get the nourishment and peace you need."

So, practice saying no once a day.

Begin in relatively safe arenas:

Say no to a friend who wants you to accompany her when what you really want to do is stay home.

Say no to a request to attend a social gathering you have no desire to attend.

Say no to your nagging inner voice that says you have to finish every last piece of work now, this very second.

Say no to eating when you are not hungry.

Saying no is a way of being tender with yourself and honest with the people around you — because if you say yes when you mean no, everyone can tell. If you say no with your voice, you will no longer need to say it with your body weight.

And when you say no to what you don't want, you can begin saying yes to what you do.

39. Be Willing to Lose the Suffering Contest

Suffering has a good name. It's hip to suffer. It's noble. It's holy. It's politically correct. And misery loves company.

A few weeks ago, I gave a lecture in San Francisco. A woman named Molly stood up and said that she had saved enough money to enable her to quit her job for the summer and travel. She also said that she planned to spend long hours doing nothing. "The problem is," she continued, "that today was the first day I didn't work and I spent the entire day eating dough-nuts. I'm panicked that by the end of the summer, I will have gained fifty pounds. That all I will do in my time off is eat."

"Why do you think you ate doughnuts today?" I asked.

"Because I felt guilty about not working. All my friends were at work. I think they are jealous of me. They think it's decadent to do nothing."

But if she suffers because she spends her time eating, they won't be jealous. If she suffers because she gains ten pounds, they won't want what she has. If she stays home all day and eats instead of getting on a plane and traveling, they can't call her "deca-dent."

The most painful part about all this is that she and her friends are on the same side. She believes that "it's wrong" to have it so easy. She believes that toiling, giving up what you want, and going without what you need builds character.

"Does that mean," I asked her, "that happiness makes you weak willed and spineless?"

"Something like that," she answered. "Also, it leaves you lonely."

Most of us are caught in this very same place without realizing it. We have moral judgments about happiness and joy. We believe that poverty, pain, and going without dessert is rewarded by God. To make matters worse, we also believe that she who does not suffer should keep her mouth shut.

With unconscious beliefs such as these, we will never let ourselves be happy. Why should we? Our friends would abandon us, we would become weak-willed sissies, and God wouldn't like it.

In a recent workshop, I asked the participants what would happen if they allowed themselves to be happy. One woman said, "I'd have to lose the suffering contest."

Yep, it's true. But when you lose this particular contest, you win something even more important: the capacity to feel delicious joy.

40. Eat Enough Protein

In my many years of teaching, writing, and listening to people talk about food, I've come to the conclusion that there are two kinds of people in the world: those who crave fat and salt, and those who crave sugar. Sometimes, but very rarely, a person is passionate about both. I know there are many reasons for this, from hormonal imbalances to allergies to yin/yang deficiencies to blood types, but it still boils down to potato chips or chocolate. If all foods were created equal, most of the thirty thousand people I've worked with over the years would throw protein out altogether.

For most of my life, I thought protein was a waste of time, calories, and taste buds. Since all I really wanted was sugar, specifically chocolate, specifically 65 percent bittersweet chocolate from France, I figured that I might as well spend my thousand calories a day on what I wanted most. This mono-food theory of eating served me well until I lost my hair, couldn't get out of bed, and realized that my internal organs were like milkweed pods in winter. Dry and shriveled.

To be honest, it wasn't the chocolate's fault. I did have some years in which I was Ms. Natural Foods. I wore Birkenstocks and ate brown rice, seaweed, and foods that most people can't pronounce. Protein was not a big part of those meals, either. Then there was the oat bran craze, the pasta craze, the eat-like-our-ancestors-who-lived-on-fruit-and-berries craze. In all of these, protein was the bad guy; if you ate too much of it, it would ferment in your intestines and your only recourse would be high colonics. Yuck.

After listening to tens of thousands of people tell me how they eat and how they feel after they eat, and after many consultations with doctors and nutritionists about my own eating habits, this is what I have learned about protein:

- ꙮ The craving for sweets is often a sign that you haven't eaten enough protein.

- ꙮ Without it, you can get very sick. What happened to me can happen to you: You can lose your bounce. Your hair can get sparse. Your nails can crack. Your skin can look gray and lifeless.

- ꙮ Your body needs protein to rebuild and repair itself.

- ꙮ Your hair, muscle, skin, nails, blood, hormones, enzymes, and brain neurotransmitters are made of protein.

- ꙮ To feel well, you must eat enough protein.

- ꙮ Consult a health professional you respect to

find out how much you need. Experiment with eating different amounts of protein. Eat the type and amount that feel best to you.

And remember: Woman cannot live on chocolate-covered potato chips alone.

41. About the Activity Formerly Known As Exercise

Rats. The "e" word again.

My friend Betty urged me not to write "one single word about exercise." She said, "We are all *sick* of hearing about the beneficial effects of aerobic activities. Be kind to your readers—forget about mentioning exercise."

I respect my friend Betty. She's wise and funny and sensitive. And she hates exercise. I followed her advice and finished the first version of the book without even mentioning the "e" word. Then, I read an article in the *San Francisco Chronicle* describing an athletic center in Los Angeles replete with treadmills and heated swimming pools, massage therapists, personal trainers, and chiropractors. This would ordinarily not be news, especially in L.A., except that its clients work out on four legs instead of two and have fur instead of hair. The header for the article read, "Why take a walk in the park when you can put your pooch on a treadmill?"

My reactions to the piece were, in this order, astonishment, laughter, and more than a spiritually correct allowance of haughty disapproval. Then, since Blanche, our cat, had an upcoming appointment with the cat chiropractor who was recommended by our veterinarian/acupuncturist, I realized I needed to lose the smugness in a hurry.

But something still troubled me. Why walk a dog on a treadmill when there are trees and paths right outside the door? Why coop her up inside when she could run outside in the sun and wind and rain? As I pondered these questions, I realized that the concept of exercising on treadmills was no more ridiculous for dogs than for humans. The whole idea that we have taken our basic, joyful impulse to move our bodies and reduced it to the drudgery of thirty-minutes-three-times-a-week exercise is crazy-making and guilt-producing. And completely disconnected from anything real.

Somewhere between the ages of seven and thirteen, we lost the connection to our bodies. We lost the sense that what was inside us mattered, and began to treat our bodies as objects that needed to be manipulated and sculpted so other people would love us. We started to diet. We started to binge. We stopped feeling the power and strength of our arms and legs and began to focus on cellulite instead.

The reason to engage in the activity formerly known as exercise is *not* because it is good for your heart or lowers your cholesterol or that your thighs are dimpled and your arms are droopy. (Most of us already know about the physical and mental benefits of exercise, but this does not seem to be enough to tear us away from the television.) The reason is *not* because you are not good enough the way you are. If you exercise for any of these reasons, your desire will last for a week, a month, maybe even a year. And then you will rebel. No one can tolerate being told they are not good enough for very long.

"Sometimes it is necessary/to reteach a thing its loveliness," writes the poet Galway Kinnell. The reason to move is to reteach our bodies their loveliness. We live most of our lives in our minds, but the fact is that we are spirits clothed in flesh and blood and bones. By not moving our bodies, we are depriving ourselves of knowing our own loveliness. We are depriving ourselves of the magnificent celebration of our own strength and power. We are depriving ourselves of reconnecting with the basic, childlike exhilaration of knowing wind and sun through the physical vehicle we were given: our bodies. We've replaced the singular, personal joy of moving outside with the grin-and-bear-it working out on machines. Yuck.

So, what to do?

Approach the "e" word with softness, humor, and care.

Stop battering, threatening, and torturing yourself.

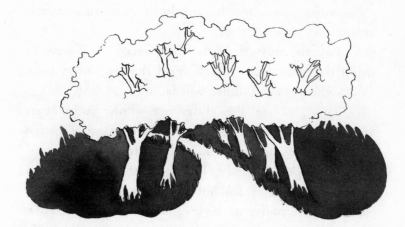

Stop whipping yourself into shape.

Understand that taking the misery (and therefore the rebellion) from exercise is a Major Big Deal because it involves unlearning self-hatred and relearning your own loveliness.

Now, take a breath, and do the following experiment:

Say to yourself, "OK, little missy—it's time to whip that butt into shape!" Feel the tension in your body when you say those words.

Then, notice the difference—how your heart opens and your muscles relax—when you say, "Listen softly, darling, I know you've been trying really hard to have a perfect body. Either that, or you've been beating yourself up for not trying hard enough. How about an alternative to the crashing and burning? How about relearning your own loveliness through the body you already have?" (Of course, your mind might be telling you that this idea of relearning loveliness is preposterous, which would have a considerable effect on the opening of your heart. If this is the case, simply notice the name-calling and let it go. If you don't pay it any attention, it will pass.)

Underneath your beliefs about the "e" word is a kid who has been cooped up inside for years and is dying to tear out of the house. She may not be the best athlete or the fastest runner or the first to get picked for the soccer team, but she still has legs to carry her in the wind, and arms to give her speed and power, and she is hungry to use them.

Imagine you are this kid. What you would do when your mother finally let you out of the house. Would you walk? Dance? Run? What is it that your body wants to do? This is not the same as what you would excel at doing.

My colleague Francie White, a dietitian whose practice focuses on resolving the causes of emotional eating and exercise resistance, says she tells people who loathe exercise to stop doing it. When they are truly ready to play, when it doesn't feel like torture or misery to move their bodies, she asks them to commit to the activities (i.e., walking outside; putting on music when no one is home and dancing around the room; Rollerblading; bicycle riding; trampoline jumping; swimming) they find most pleasurable five days a week.

For the rest of their lives.

I ask my students to do the same.

The reason the commitment is important is because even after you've rediscovered the joy and power of moving your arms and legs, you still have to endure a whole lifetime, and the entire fitness industry, pushing you in the direction of exercise-as-suffering, exercise-for-results. Without a firm commitment, you will waver. You will think you are not working hard enough. You will believe that true happiness can only come from a culturally perfect body, and since you probably don't have one, you will doubt your experience.

The new ads for The Body Shop say, "There are three billion women who don't look like super models and only eight who do." In the end, moving your body is not about flat stomachs or thin thighs; it is about being one of the three billion women on the planet who is lucky enough to have arms and legs that can surge with energy, be warmed by the sun, and slice through wind and water. Moving your body is about physically connecting with the fundamental joy and gratitude of being alive. The rest is gravy.

42. Take the Woo-Woo Out of Meditation

To meditate, you don't have to wear red dots on your forehead, say Indian-sounding mantras, or hold your fingers in funny positions. You don't have to sit on a special cushion, cross your legs, or burn incense. Most especially, you can meditate and still be passionate about retail therapy, crunchy cheese sticks, and Erica on *All My Children*.

I've been meditating for twenty-two years and have had no mystical experiences, no altered states, no visions of light or angels. The reason I continue to meditate is because it is a way of settling, a way of landing in myself, of being present. I meditate because when I do, I feel complete.

My friend Caitriona Reed, a meditation teacher in San Diego, says, "When we learn to meditate, we are learning to become whole, aware, alive, well. All these words apply, but they still infer there is something we lack which meditation can give us. It might be easier if we understood that meditation does not give us anything at all, rather it removes the obstacles that prevent us from being whole.

"Practicing mindfulness, we discover that the way we live this moment, for example, will affect the whole day, our whole life. If we can bring awareness to this moment, there is happiness, not through the fulfillment of desires, but simply because awareness is there. Simply to see, hear, touch, know — a tree, a street corner, a person — is its own reward. The rest of the day will be altered. Simple as it is, our capacity just to be attentive is the vital key to our happiness."

If this is really true, if it were possible to be happy simply by being attentive, wouldn't it be worth the effort? If the reason you want to be thin, rich, or in love is to be happy, and if you could be happy this very moment without having to be thin or rich or in love, wouldn't it be worth a try?

You have nothing to lose except twenty minutes a day in which you would otherwise be rushing around trying to get to the next place so that you could finally feel what you would feel if you sat in one place.

Set aside twenty minutes before you start your day. Sit in a chair with your back straight and relaxed, and both feet on the floor. Let your breathing become easy, soft. Now, become aware of an area about three inches below your navel. Focus on that area. Count to ten. If your mind wanders, start again. When you reach ten, start at one.

If you take less than twenty minutes, you won't give your attention a chance to settle. Our lives move so quickly that when we sit down, we are like lakes during a summer storm. Ruffled, agitated, cloudy. When you breathe for twenty minutes, you give the weather a chance to move through. You become still, calm, centered, clear.

After that, you're ready for anything.

43. Burn Your Diet Books in Your Bathtub and Other Rituals

∞

Some teachers recommend rituals such as lighting candles and dancing; some suggest drumming or chanting or gathering friends in the forest. Not me. I recommend that you take every single piece of diet junk you've collected, toss it into your bathtub in the middle of the afternoon, and gleefully set it ablaze.

Why such boldness? Such aggression? Such pyromania?

Because it is a proclamation of freedom from the

voice inside that believes that one day, when your life has calmed down a bit and the kids have gone to college and your life is just the way you want it to be, you will look like the leotard-clad models in the tummy-flattener articles. The boldness of this decision and the courage it takes to make it deserve a grand gesture. They deserve a parade, a standing ovation, Liberace playing "Hail to the Queen" on the piano. But since parades and standing ovations are probably not available, and since Liberace died years ago, setting a small, contained bonfire within six inches of a water faucet seems like a respectable second choice.

I speak from experience.

One of the very first things I did twenty years ago when I decided I would no longer diet was to collect every scrap of diet riffraff I'd accumulated and burn it in my bathtub. Sandwiching the articles between the books, I struck a kitchen match, and watched it all burn. After that, there was no going back. I had cleansed my desk, bookshelves, and mind of the idea that a better life was waiting for me around the corner if I could only become a different, thinner person.

When I burned my diet books, I told myself that I was burning the idea that if I could only deprive myself enough, whip myself into shape, I would have the life I knew was possible. The fire cleansed the past, made room for the present.

In my workshops, I recommend burning diet books or creating other bold rituals that can be imprinted in your memory and used as touchstones of strength. They need to be bold because the gremlin in your head that says "You can't, you mustn't, you won't, it's impossible, not now, not for twenty years . . ." has claws, tentacles, suckers, and a thousand arms to strangle you. Outrageous, bold acts that don't hurt anyone, including yourself (putting your scale through the trash compactor and making bird food out of your diet bars are other examples), evoke heart, courage, and intention, which are different, but equally powerful, kinds of strength.

This is part of a letter I received from a student who attended a recent workshop: "I walked into the class on Friday and sat down. Tears came to my eyes. You got up and said, 'Hello. I'm Geneen Roth,' and the torrent started. I tried to stop crying, but I couldn't. I felt like such a fool. God, I was afraid I would be thrown out. I was afraid people would laugh at me, I was afraid that I was going to find out I really wasn't worth anything. That I really didn't matter at all. And that all the pain I was feeling was unfounded and self-ish. That I had no right to want love and care from other people. I almost ran out of the room.

"During the first small group, I told four total strangers about my past. They responded with concern and sympathy. I still don't believe it. When strangers said, 'You have every right to your pain,' I couldn't put it into words. This is what I have been hoping for all my life. This was the greatest risk I have ever taken and it came out all right.

"I returned to my house with a plan I lifted from you. First I cleaned my apartment. I collected every secret piece of diet paraphernalia I had. I took the pile out to my hibachi grill on my front porch. I got the idea from the fact that you burned your diet books in your bathtub. But my bathtub is plastic, and California is always in danger of burning down, so I figured my

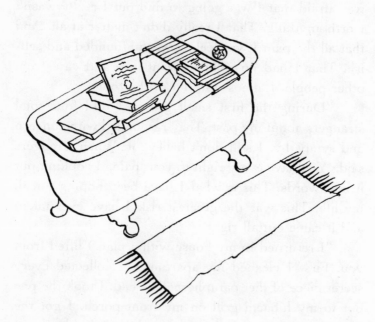

little grill was the safest place to have a bold ritual. I started the fire with the torn pages of *Thirty Days to Thinner Thighs* and dumped the remains of my jar of California Slim into the fire. I kept it going with pages I had torn out of *Mademoiselle* and *Glamour* and *Self*. The pages filled with diet and exercise tips (most of it unread), the pages of the models I wanted to look like, the pages of the bodies I dreamed of having. One by one, I threw the remaining Dexatrim pills into the fire and continued feeding pages to keep the fire alive. I reached my emotional peak the moment I began tearing up the latest copy of *Cosmopolitan* and feeding it to the flames.

"Unfortunately, the Ultra Slim-Fast bars I was also burning created a lot of smoke and a pretty bad stench, and my female neighbor (a California blonde who lives in an aerobics studio) ran out to the porch and called to my male neighbor (whose second home is the gym), 'Do you smell something burning? Is the apartment on fire?'

"I was behind a narrow partition and stuck my head out and said, 'No, no, it's just me. I'm finally using my hibachi.' They came over to look at the flames while I tried to hide the crumpled pages of the latest *Cosmo* Quiz on "Does he *really* love you?" under my legs and they asked what I was cooking. I couldn't think fast enough and said, 'Oh, I'm not cooking anything. I'm just getting rid of a few things.' They eyed each other suspiciously and the male neighbor remarked that that was an interesting way to spend the evening.

"When the ashes were cool enough to be sifted through with my hands, I scooped them into a bag and drove to the park. I walked to a particularly beautiful spot and scattered the ashes in the wind. I went back home and cooked a wonderful meal for myself—cream of zucchini soup, broiled salmon steak, scalloped potatoes, asparagus, and for dessert, cognac and chocolate truffles. I'm a wonderful cook, and this is the first time I have ever made anything for myself. But it won't be the last."

Burning your diet books doesn't itself create change; it is a bridge, a signal, a wild, outrageous act that underscores your intention to free yourself from the ways you confine yourself, punish yourself, hate yourself. Burning your diet books is like jumping into a plane and swooping around the sky, writing, "I am free! I am free! I am free!" in letters as big as buildings. After you get out of the plane, you still have to pay attention to the ways you aren't free, you still have to act on your own behalf with curiosity and kindness, you still have to live your life. But bold, symbolic acts create bridges upon which you can take the first few steps. They also provide an outlet for the very same energy that fuels a binge — immense, powerful, creative energy that has been imprisoned in years of dieting. So, what are you waiting for?

44. Do One Exquisitely Kind Thing for Yourself Every Day

My friend Barbara used to say, "What most people consider necessities, I consider irrelevant. What most people consider luxuries, I consider necessities." Barbara knew how to be kind to herself. She painted her house in soft, enveloping colors, took a peach bubble bath every night, spent time outdoors every day. When she had two children, she still managed to do one thing a day just for herself. Even for fifteen minutes.

Most women consider being kind to themselves a luxury, not a necessity. Like Barbara, I maintain that it is a necessity.

To break out of the habitual and unkind ways we feel about ourselves, we have to create new habits. We have to treat ourselves with unaccustomed grace. With kindness, tenderness, and a great deal of humor. In the beginning, this will seem alternately frivolous and difficult. It will seem like too much trouble. But remember that treating yourself unkindly is also a habit; in the beginning, it was painful to be mean to yourself, but you've done it so many times that it's now effortless.

Keep in mind that children will not be naturally unkind to themselves.

It takes time to learn to deprive yourself.

It also takes great effort to become effortless at anything. And it takes just as much effort to be mean as to be kind. So why not expend your energy on cultivating kindness?

Here are some suggestions of ways to be kind to yourself to which you can add your own:

Do One Exquisitely Kind Thing for Yourself Every Day

꙰ Paint a wall of your home in a color that you could go swimming in. Drink in the color.

꙰ Do absolutely nothing for fifteen minutes.

꙰ Go into the bathroom, lock the door, and read.

꙰ Throw out your underwear with holes and stains.

꙰ Buy new underwear.

꙰ Say you are sorry to someone you have been wanting to say you are sorry to for a long, long time.

꙰ Take a sledgehammer to your scale.

45. When Diets Do Work

I know I've spent a hundred pages telling you why diets don't work. But since there *really* is no one right way (see chapter 21), I would be lying by omission if I didn't tell you when they do.

When I was thirty-five, I was diagnosed with shingles. For the next seven years, I was ill, with constant diarrhea and a series of viruses, from pneumonia to pleurisy to flus. I felt like a string of antique pearls — fragile, brittle, always in danger of shattering. None of the twenty doctors or healers I consulted could tell me what was wrong. During the worst of it, I lost my hair, my skin broke out in bleeding rashes, and my fingernails fell off.

Then I met a doctor who, after a series of blood tests, put me on a diet. Since I'd been sick, other doctors had prescribed diets—yeast-free, high-protein, macrobiotic—and I had tried them all, but they didn't work. I felt the way I always felt on diets: crazed, deprived, and out of control. Every one of those diets would be followed by a knock-your-socks-off binge. (As sick as I was, I never lost my verve for bingeing after a diet.) But this diet was different because it made sense; it was aligned with my soul. By that I mean that if I had been able to push past my shticks about food, I would have already known, and already been doing, what this doctor told me to do.

During our first visit, she said, "Think of your body as the earth. If you want to plant a life-giving garden, you need to make sure the soil is loamy and rich with nutrients. For most of your life, you've stripped the ground and still expected to grow healthy plants. Now, you need to put some minerals back.

"Eat less sugar and starch. Eat more protein, and more fat. Eat snacks, even at bedtime. Move your body every day. Use nature as a restorative. Rest twice as much as you already do."

After she spoke, I felt as if the cells in my body stood up and cheered, "Finally! Someone is talking sense to this girl!" But what came out of my mouth was, "I can't do this. I will get fat." My doctor said, "I don't think you will — your body is starved for this kind of nourishment — but what would you rather have? A ragged, hairless, thin body or a healthy, radiant, bigger body?"

It was, as they say, "a moment."

Matt was sitting beside me, waiting to hear the answer. I'm sure he was astonished that I was actually considering the question, and was wondering if he had married a lunatic. I knew I had no choice, but I also knew that if I started this "diet" I had to be willing to gain weight, possibly ten or twenty pounds. I had to become a beginner again, throw out the no-diet expert image, start over.

Which is exactly what I did. For the first two months, I was tentative, fearful, and wacky. I kept calling the doctor with questions: Why do I need so much protein? What about all these studies that say that needing a lot of protein is a myth, not to mention harmful for the kidneys? What about fat being bad for the heart?

"Some people," she said, "don't need as much protein; some people don't need as much fat. But, given your history and blood test results, you need more of both."

Seventeen years of fasting followed by overeating followed by dieting on Grape-Nuts or cigarettes and Diet Shasta creme soda had taken their toll. At eleven, when I should have been making sure I was getting enough calcium to create strong bones, I was going on my first diet. At fifteen, when I should have been eating enough protein and fat to sustain the feverish pace of adolescence, I started a four-year stint of diet pills. At twenty-five, I was anorexic. At twenty-seven, I gained eighty pounds in two months. And although my body had done a superb job of supporting me despite unremitting negligence — my legs had climbed mountains, my hands had written books, my heart had never stopped beating, opening, loving—it was, as Andy Griffith used to say, "just plum wore out." Because, though it appeared as if I were feeding my body, I'd been feeding my mind, my past wounds, my present stress.

I've been on this "diet" for four years now. I gained five pounds in the first three months, and although I panicked at the beginning of the weight gain, I stayed uncharacteristically clear that my priority was being strong and well. "If I have to be fat," I kept saying to myself, "I will be." Six months later, my body adjusted to the new way of eating, and I lost the weight.

Sometimes I eat more sugar than is best, sometimes I don't follow the instructions at all, but I know what my body needs and how to provide it. When I feel exhausted and weak, I know what to do to feel better. I will never have the robust health of someone who didn't gain and lose a thousand pounds, but if I am mindful of what I put into my body, I thrive.

The story has two morals (and neither one of

them is to eat what I eat or find out the name of my doctor!). The first is that what we do to our body has consequences. I thought I got away with the month-long water fasts followed by weeks of eating nothing but Krispy Kreme doughnuts. But all those years of emotional eating had their effect: My health is fragile, I have gone though premature, illness-induced menopause, and I've been diagnosed with osteoporosis.

If, when I was eleven, someone had told me that the way I was eating might cripple me at age sixty, I probably would have kept right on eating Oreos for breakfast. And at age twenty, nutritional guidance probably wouldn't have stopped me from raw-food diets and the ensuing anorexia. Nevertheless, I still wish someone had told me; I wish I could have made an informed choice about the food I ate and the course I was charting for the rest of my life.

So, I'll be the one to say it now: What you eat matters, not only to the size of your body but to its well-being. Depending on the strength of your constitution, your genetic background, your environment, and your inner life, the food you eat will skew your biochemistry in a particular direction, which will then affect the course of your life. This is not a prediction or a fear-based assumption; it is simply cause and effect.

The second moral is that if you need food for emotional reasons right now—and cannot tolerate the thought of monitoring kinds and amounts of proteins, fats, and sugars—it does not mean that you are crazy, wrong, and will get cancer in five years. If you start monitoring your food intake before you are ready, you will sabotage yourself again and again by bingeing. But that doesn't mean giving yourself permission to be unconscious. It doesn't mean eating everything you want whenever you want it.

Your job is to do your best at all times. To be curious, to treat yourself with kindness, and to act on your own behalf. You need to know when to act and when to reflect, when to push and when to let go. Your job is to keep an open and tender heart and to be aware of your limits. The time will come, if it hasn't already, when for you right action—action that is aligned with your soul—will be to be discriminating about the kinds and amounts of foods you put into the soil of your body. This is the time when the kind of diet I am referring to in this chapter works. And you'll know it's right because you won't feel as if all the sweetness in the world has just been ripped out from under your feet. You won't feel as if you are being deprived of the goodies in life. It won't be hard, which isn't to say that it won't take effort; it always takes effort to learn new practices. But it's a different kind of effort from the usual diet, which entails punishing and being at war with yourself on a daily basis.

When does a diet work?

When it doesn't feel like a diet.

When your body sings in response to the discriminations you make in the foods you eat. And when listening to that body song is a priority. Most of the time.

When you are willing to choose foods that support your highest, clearest, light-giving self. Most of the time.

When saying no to particular foods feels as if you are blessing yourself with vitality and energy rather than depriving yourself of fried onion rings. Most of the time.

When you understand that when it's not most of the time, doing your best is eating ice cream for breakfast and the hell with everything else.

46. Consider Resigning from Your Fondness for Drama

Telling yourself you are fat is fabulous drama. So is telling yourself you are ugly, dumb, incompetent, and worthless. Besides being dramatic, it is also time-consuming and anxiety-producing. You can spend your whole life bouncing back and forth between extremes of dramatic, agitating feelings. Most of us do. Like people who need to place themselves in physical danger to feel fully alive, most of us find that drama and agitation are strong, enlivening positions. You cannot be numb and agitated at the same time. You don't feel dead when you are famished, miserable, worthless.

As I mentioned at the beginning of this book, sometimes, in a workshop, I ask: "What would your life be like if you woke up tomorrow and suddenly didn't have a problem with food?" For people who don't have issues with food, the question is still the same. What would you do and think about if the main problem of your life was suddenly gone?

At first, most people smile. Ahhhh. To wake up and be thin. To wake up and feel brilliant. To wake up and be in love. How divine. What could be wrong with that? Then, reality sets in. But what would I do all day long? What would I think about?

Then they say:

"I think I would be bored."

"I'd have to deal with my loveless marriage."

"I wouldn't know myself without this problem."

The drama itself is incredibly alluring, and seductive. It's not that feeling fat feels good; we all know it feels terrible. But at least it feels like *something*. It also feels familiar and, therefore, comforting. Feeling fat or ugly or dumb is its own complete world. To give it up you must first understand that it has been providing you with a focus and a whipped-up kind of excitement.

Imagine what your life would be like without the drama of feeling fat. What would change? What would you notice that you don't notice now?

What would it be like to be hungry without being famished, to be sad without being devastated, to see what's there without adding dramatic flourishes?

What would it be like to eat a lot, to be so full that you can't move and *not* feel that you are seconds away from being as big as a house? To understand that sometimes everyone overeats?

How would your definition of yourself change?

What would you do with all the time that you used to spend worrying about your weight and feeling fat?

These are burning questions. Live with them, turn them over. Wrestle with the answers. If you don't have answers, keep asking the questions. Sometimes, just asking the questions is enough to turn around your mind, to turn around your heart.

If you weren't convinced you were fat or ugly, who would you be?

47. Food and Your Mother Go Together

We first knew we were loved by getting held and fed by our mothers. In those days, food *was* love. Mother was love. Our whole life depended on one person and on her ability to feed us. And although we are grown-ups now, these ancient connections are still stored in our bodies and minds. The issue with food is love and sweetness. The issue with mother is love and sweetness. The issues about being alive are often the many ways we experience and are deprived of love and sweetness.

When I despair about getting caught in the same

old mother-loss issues — the feelings of abandonment, the longing for unconditional love, the belief that I am damaged at my core, the intense hunger for sweetness in the form of ice cream and chocolate — my meditation teacher says, "Only people who are dead or enlightened are finished with the stuff about their mothers." And that always makes me feel better about being miserable.

I used to think it was possible to be done forever with emotional eating. I don't believe that anymore. (That is not the same as believing it is a disease; I don't believe that either.) While my weight has fluctuated only by four or five pounds in nearly twenty years, I've realized that I will probably use food in one way or another until I know for absolutely certain that I am lovable, that my truest, deepest nature is love. I hope this happens soon, but if it doesn't, if there are moments when I turn to food for love, then all I need to do is pay attention, and be curious, kind, and willing to act on my own behalf. I need to ask myself what is really going on, and then I need to do something about it.

Food and mothers go together even for people who haven't habitually turned to food for comfort. My friend Daisy is not an emotional eater. Food has never been a problem for her. In fact, being skinny has been her problem. This was a major stumbling block for me when we met. Not that there's anything wrong with being skinny your whole life, but REALLY. It seemed like such a waste of my hard-earned insight to be friends with someone who couldn't appreciate a good binge or my extensive research on the best sweet potato pie in San Francisco. I soon realized, however, that while I was developing my food skills, she was developing her shopping skills, and that between the two, we pretty much had the material world covered.

Anyway, Daisy recently uncovered some early feelings she had in relation to her mother, who had been dead for ten years. And what do you think she did? At one sitting, she ate a whole rhubarb pie. At another, a pint of Ben & Jerry's New York Super Fudge Chunk. There was something about feeling the loss of that sweet, merging, mother connection that made her want to eat. She gained five pounds in eight days. I told her I had a few good books to recommend. . . .

My students often say, "I want to be done with this thing with food once and for all." But there is no place to get to, no such thing as arriving and never having to leave. If you take a big view and understand that eating, or thinking about eating, will probably always be the way you alert yourself to changes in your inner world, you can relax. You can use turning to food as a method of exploring the corners of your soul; you can think about emotional eating as a gift rather than a curse.

Ask yourself what you want from being alive. If the answer is that you want "She Was Thin" engraved on your headstone, then forget what I am saying. Lose weight at any cost.

If what you want is to know all the folded-down corners of yourself, to understand why you do the things you do and to use your experiences as a road map, then it's okay to relax.

The way to enlightenment is paved with good food and silky clothes. My mother told me so.

48. Separate the Desire to Be Thin from the Desire to Be Cherished

When I first started teaching, a student came to my class after she'd lost a hundred pounds on a fast and had gained fifty of it back. "They lied to me," she said. "They said my life would be great when I got thin. They said I would be happy. They said I would love myself. They said I would be loved. But that's not what happened. Sure, I liked being thin. I liked wearing smaller clothes. I liked feeling lighter. But changing my outside didn't change my inside. I still felt like a fat person — unworthy, unlovable, damaged. I was so disappointed, and felt so betrayed by everyone, beginning with my parents, who had always promised that things would change when I got thin, that I started to eat again."

In *Into Thin Air*, a book about the 1996 Mt. Everest disaster, Jon Krakauer describes his lifelong dream of climbing the famous mountain. From the time he was nine, he says he lived to climb. When he finally made it to the summit, he found himself "atop a slender wedge of ice, adorned with a discarded oxygen cylinder and a battered aluminum survey pole, with nowhere higher to climb.

"Reaching the top of Everest is supposed to trigger a surge of intense elation: against all odds, after all, I had just attained a goal I'd coveted since childhood. But the summit is really only the halfway point.... I stayed on top of the world just long enough to fire off four quick [photographic] shots. Then I turned to descend."

You dream of being thin, you work hard at it, you postpone your other dreams, certain that when you get there, the struggle will have been worth it. Then, at last, you find yourself there . . . but the top of the world is just another place. A wedge of time, a body size, that's all. Being thin is only the halfway point. You have to keep moving, eating, living.

This lack of finality, the fact that the relationship with food and body size is an ongoing process, not an end point, a place at which you arrive and from which everything looks different, is the most difficult, most painful, and most elusive insight to sustain. Even people who lose weight five, ten, twenty times and gain it back continue to believe that next time, it will be different. Next time, they will keep it off. Next time, being thin will finally fulfill its promise of everlasting happiness. Being thin always seems to be synonymous with happiness, joy, self-worth, and love despite the fact that it cannot possibly provide these things.

If it's happiness you want, why not go directly to it? Why not put your energy and attention there rather than on the size of your body? Why not look inside rather than outside? Why continue to climb Mt. Everest when the view is also breathtaking from the hill down the block?

Which is not to say that you should accept being

fat. Attaining your natural weight is a fine goal. Besides making life easier by allowing you to fit into the cultural standard, losing weight also enables you to be more physical, take stress off your heart and joints, choose from a wide variety of clothes, fit into one chair. There are many good reasons to be thin, but being cherished should not be one of them. Because it won't work. Being cherished and the size of your body are not related—you only believe they are. The truth is that you deserve to be cherished and to cherish yourself *no matter what you weigh.*

The bad news is that being thin is not going to do what you think it's going to do. If it did, everyone who is now or has ever been thin would be happy.

And the good news is that you can have whatever you believe being thin will give you, and you can have it now.

How can you have it? By living as if you liked yourself. By not tolerating fat-and-ugly attacks. By making a commitment to be kind to yourself and not letting anything stand in your way. By setting aside time for yourself daily. By believing that what you do, you do for good reasons, and by being curious about what those reasons are. By being vigilant about acting on your own behalf. By doing—not just thinking about—the suggestions in this book. By beginning today. By understanding that in reading this book and coming this far, you already have.

49. Celebrate Every Little Thing

ھ

I call Sally my "what-the-hell" friend because she uses any reason to celebrate. Every dinner is a cause to break out her good silver. She paints each toenail a different color and wears eyeglasses that glitter. We drink water from crystal goblets her grandmother gave her. Even when her three-year-old son, sixty-pound shaggy dog, and two cats are running around, she uses her best dishes. No matter how I feel when I arrive at her house I soon find myself thinking, "Oh, what the hell. Might as well drink champagne. Might as well paint my toenails gold. Might as well take a bath in the middle of the day in her giant tub with the mermaid soap dish. What was I so caught up in before I got here, anyway?" Her attitude is "Create feasts. Make noises. Celebrate every little thing," and when I am with her, I do.

I had a boyfriend once who didn't love me. Usually, I am so humiliated by the memory of how I threw myself at his feet that I either repress everything he ever said to me, or else portray him to readers as heartless and ignorant (revenge being one of a writer's great advantages). But this morning, as I was thinking about celebrating every little thing, I suddenly recalled something he said during a fight we had at Greens Restaurant in San Francisco. "Why not think of all the times we've celebrated and all the times we have yet to celebrate as a bank account from which we can draw funds?" he asked. "Let's take some celebration savings out now, put aside this fight, and replenish the fund when we get home. How about it?" I remember looking from him to the cheese and mushroom tart on my plate, thinking, "I could let this horrible fight go. The churning in my stomach could stop, I could enjoy this tart, and we could have a wonderful time." Then I thought, "But if I let it go, I'll be a wimp, a chump, a pushover. He doesn't deserve to have a good time after what he did." I figured that if he didn't love me, the least he could do was suffer. So I said, "Forget it. It's a terrible idea," and ruined the evening for us both.

It's taken me thirteen years to remember that I was enchanted by the notion of a celebration fund, and to admit that even cads can have brilliant ideas. Drawing from celebration savings is a way of contacting the part of our beings that is like an ongoing parade. Or a dazzling clear-blue sky. It is like taking off in an airplane during a rainstorm, and flying above the clouds. You suddenly realize that this luminous blue has been there all the time. When you draw from a celebration fund, you set aside your involvement with your drama-of-the-moment and contact the exhilarating spaciousness beneath it. And you can do this whenever you want! It is like having Christmas in the middle of July, or your birthday on any day you choose.

The idea of a celebration fund is related to labeling, one of the first meditation techniques I ever learned. When you notice you are thinking, label it "thinking." Don't get involved in the content—who did what to whom, what you are going to do about it, etc. No matter how compelling the thought is, no matter how urgent it seems, every time you notice you're thinking, simply label it and let the thought go.

The object of labeling is twofold: First, as I mentioned earlier, is understanding that there is no solid or meaningful basis for our thoughts. They have no apparent beginning or end. The mind is like a wind-up toy that never winds down. And while it is necessary to be able to think, it is a huge relief to have a way to get out from under the constant whir of thoughts. Labeling enables you to wrap up a thought, tie it in a bow, and let it go. When the next thought comes, you label it "thinking," and in so doing, let go of it as well. After a while, you realize that thoughts just keep coming, and as you keep labeling them, they pass by without seducing you into the whos, whats, and whens.

The second benefit of labeling is that when you

disengage from the white noise of your thoughts, you feel a sense of pure and delicious freedom. Pema Chödrön, a Tibetan Buddhist teacher, likens being caught in your thinking to sitting in front of the Grand Canyon with a bag on your head. When you label your thoughts, you lift the bag off your head and arrive in the present moment (see chapter 10), giving yourself a chance to celebrate the sheer fact of being alive. We are usually so identified with our story lines that we do not even consider who we are apart from them; we do not realize that we are not our thoughts.

Sometimes, when you are walking along the street caught in your story line of the moment (what happened yesterday, what you need to do tomorrow, what you wish you had said to the guy who insulted you at the bank), you catch sight of something that makes you stop thinking. A child with red, curly hair trying to train her new puppy. A row of giant coral dahlias. A mime who has sprayed himself silver and looks exactly like the Tin Man in *The Wizard of Oz*. And suddenly, whatever was going on before seems silly and small and irrelevant, and you are sublimely happy. That is the moment when you realize that you are so much bigger than your thoughts. You feel like celebrating for no reason at all except that the sun is out and the color coral exists and the traffic light turned green, and you are a part of the ongoing wonder and the wonder is part of you.

Unless you are Sally-like and find celebrating life effortless, I recommend following these three steps to remind yourself that if it's worth doing, it's worth celebrating:

1. Use labeling as a way to disengage yourself from the seriousness of your own stories. I practice labeling not only when I meditate, but when I am any-where—walking along a street, hiking in the forest, riding on an airplane, being with a friend—and feel as if I have a bag over my head. (Usually, this is at least once every day.)

2. Seize every excuse to celebrate. You woke up today. Your hair is clean. You ate when you were hungry. The wind is ruffling the leaves on the trees. You have arms and legs.

3. When all else fails, and you have an irresistible urge for revenge during a time of festivity, draw on the celebration fund. Learn from my experience with the cad: Don't miss the mushroom tarts of your life.

My accountant has a poster in her office of a bald, eighty-year-old man in a black leather jacket on a motorcycle. It says "Work hard and save all your money so that when you are old, you can afford things that only young people enjoy."

In case you need a boost, here are some ideas for how to celebrate, just for the hell of it: Paint stars on your ceiling; make noises when you eat; put a clown nose on when you drive; wear a flower behind your ear; light candles every night; send yourself (or anyone else) a bouquet of yellow tulips; use your best dishes every day, especially when you eat in front of the refrigerator.

One more thing: Celebrate what you have before you are too old and cranky to enjoy it. Get that black leather jacket today.

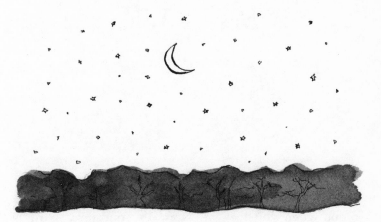

Celebrate Every Little Thing

50. Decide on an Everyday Practice and Do It No Matter What

We've come to the end of the book. I've told you every-thing I know about feeling thin and happy and gor-geous when you feel fat. Now it's your turn. Now is the time for insight to be put into action, and kindness and curiosity to be combined with acting on your own behalf.

There is no magic. No one is going to hand you the answer because *they don't have it.* You do. But it's not going to appear in front of you like a vision, like

Acknowledgments

To:
Hameed Ali, Jeanne Hay, Alia Johnson, and my small group; Sally McCartin; Judah Betz; Premsiri Lewen; Jace Schinderman; Richard Glantz; Laurie Abkemeier, Lisa Kitei, Brian DeFiore, Kris Kliemann, and Bob Miller at Hyperion; Annie Lamott; Natalie Goldberg; Angela Miller; P. Tulip; Maureen Nemeth; Blanche, of course, and my beloved husband, Matt Weinstein.

A thousand peonies of thanks.

the prince we always dreamed about. When asked who saved her, the eight-year-old heroine in Anna Quindlen's fairy tale, *Happily Ever After*, says, "I rescued myself."

You can do it. You can rescue yourself. No matter how miserable or fat or ugly you feel, no matter what you believe about your competence or your worth or your capacity to love and be loved, you can change. It doesn't matter whether you weigh four hundred pounds on the bathroom scale or inside your mind, you can become someone who knows without a doubt that she is powerful and strong and gorgeous. You can stop following the instructions you were given ten or twenty or fifty years ago. You can become every courageous inch of yourself. You can become your own heroine, but you have to act. It's up to you. No book, no teacher, no lover, no child, no God can do this for you.

Pick a practice, any practice. Read through the book and find a practice you know you can commit yourself to on a daily basis. I recommend doing something quiet and alone every morning. It could be sensing your arms and legs or sitting for twenty minutes a day or spending a half hour doing a Curiosity Dialogue.

An everyday practice allows the part of you that is not caught up in the drama of fat and ugly to show up. Otherwise, the demands of your work, your children, your busy life will crowd you out.

The most important thing is that you start acting on your own behalf, that you begin to understand that you are capable of so much more greatness that you ever imagined.

If you do not feed this part of you, it will not grow.

Some mornings will come and you will feel grumpy or tired or rushed or stressed and having a root canal will sound better than doing your practice. Do it anyway. If it means waking up at six instead of six-thirty, set the alarm for six. If it means leaving a party before they cut the cake, leave anyway. If it means not having dessert or a second cup of coffee or watching the end of the movie, do it anyway. You are working against a lifetime of not being your friend. Soon it will get easier, and then effortless. After a while, feeling fat and ugly, and turning to food to soothe yourself, will seem strange, distant, and unappealing. It will lose its hold on you.

When you're convinced you're the only one in the world who is getting up at six to do your everyday practice and still can't fit into her loose jeans, remember me. I'm right here, in my own house, doing the same thing. Let me know how it goes.

For a schedule of workshops, or information about audio and videotapes, please write:

Breaking Free
P.O. Box 2852
Santa Cruz, California, 95063
phone: (408) 685-8601
fax: (408) 685-8602

You can also visit our website @ www.geneenroth.com

About the Author

Geneen Roth is the author of five best-selling books, including *When Food is Love, Feeding the Hungry Heart, Appetites, Breaking Free from Compulsive Eating,* and *Why Weight?* A pioneer in the anti-diet movement, Roth teaches workshops across the country to help men and women understand and change their approach to food and weight issues. She lives in northern California with her husband Matt, and Blanche, the male cat, whose prodigious size has never—not for even a day—disturbed his self-esteem.